PSYCHOLOGICAL ASSESSMENT

IN MANAGED CARE

PSYCHOLOGICAL ASSESSMENT
IN MANAGED CARE

CHRIS E. STOUT

JOHN WILEY & SONS, INC.
New York • Chichester • Weinheim • Brisbane • Singapore • Toronto

Library of Congress Cataloging-in-Publication Data:
Stout, Chris E.
    Psychological assessment in managed care / by Chris E. Stout.
        p.   cm.
    Includes bibliographical references and index.
    ISBN 0-471-17033-X (cloth : alk. paper)
    1. Clinical psychology—Practice.   2. Managed mental health care.
3. Psychological tests.   I. Title.
RC467.95.S76   1997
616.89'075—dc21   96-45264

Printed in the United States of America

10   9   8   7   6   5   4   3   2   1

Preface

IN THE MANY BOOKS ON the "how-tos" of dealing with managed care, little is written for the specialty of testing and assessment. Most of this book deals with testing, assessment, and systems from a psychologist's perspective. However, other assessment concerns within managed care inevitably cross into the domain of other practitioners—primary care physicians, researchers, administrators, evaluators (vis-à-vis outcome instruments), psychiatrists, social workers, and various other users of screening instruments, surveys, and expeditious data-collecting tools.

This book neither criticizes nor champions the impact managed care has had on behavioral healthcare practice. Instead, it focuses on various means and methods of using testing and assessment activities to improve one's practice within a managed care environment.

The book's approach is pragmatic and utilitarian. It is designed, written, and meant to be used as a tool for reference, planning, and marketing.

Practice and Instruction Shifts

My academic/clinical experience partially led to this work's existence. In my own clinical practice, I have found it increasingly difficult to be able to provide psychodiagnostic consulting and assessment services within the constrictions of third-party payments and fourth-party reviewer limitations or prohibitions. Colleagues whose practices were more specialized and were solely based on assessment services had even more difficulties. I have been teaching objective assessment techniques to doctoral-level graduate students within an APA-approved program. My lectures on how to select testing instruments, as a basis for possible referral, were beginning to be amended to include a discussion of methods of gaining preapprovals, justifying test selections to fourth-party reviewers for approval, and other such new "technical" activities resulting from managed care's impact. Students' questions concerning reimbursement levels were historically answered with a statement of a range of a few hundred dollars, based on reasonable and customary charges. The only "complication" to this straightforward billing procedure would be the occasional co-pay. Today, I punctuate lectures with variations on the theme ". . . but, within a managed care environment, . . .". There is certainly nothing wrong with this per se, but although it is a practical reality in most clinicians' practices, it is often ignored in graduate instruction.

The Merit of Testing?

These and similar circumstances led to the genesis of this book, irrespective of the "academic support" of the value and merit of projective psychological testing techniques argued by Piotrowski (1984) and, more recently, by Watkins and his coauthors, that ". . . [projectives] are here to stay . . . and their place in clinical assessment practice now seems as strong as, if not stronger than, ever" (Watkins, Campbell, Nieberding, & Hallmark, 1995, p. 59). Earlier critiques (Pruitt, Smith, Thelen, & Lubin, 1985; Thelen, Varble, & Johnson, 1968) cast doubt on the longevity of the projective testing within clinical psychology. The current applied clinical atmosphere does not bode well for such testing and makes studies on the utilization of psychological testing difficult to generalize to managed care settings, if not moot. Whether one "likes" managed care or not, it is a reality now and it is likely to penetrate practices further. This is not a book to rally the troops nor an attempt to collectively bargain for assessment. I have not written a guerrilla manual on how to "work the system" of managed care. This is a broad-based but direct and realistic collection of means, methods, and ideas on how to work to maintain, if not expand, the utility and role of a variety of types of assessments in a managed care environment, in order to provide better care to patients while demonstrating psychology's key utility.

Overview

This book canvases the various areas of psychological testing and other forms of patient data collection within the context of managed care. Chapter 1 reviews the basics and the evolution of managed care, and Chapter 2 examines the role and function of family practice physicians, primary care physicians, internists, and general practitioners as "screeners" for psychopathology and identifiers of patients in need of testing services. Often, individuals will present to these medical practitioners with vague physical complaints that are actually secondary to or symptomatic of psychological disorders. To deliver the most efficient and effective level of care, medical generalists must have screening tools and psychological consultation. Psychologists must train them in the "how tos" of conveying findings to the patient and/or the family, and managing the referral most appropriately. Instruments that would be helpful to these ends are discussed.

Medical patient populations that tend to be the domain of specialists are discussed in Chapter 3, along with various strategies for providing differential diagnosis in biological cases; disorders that mimic psychological malingering cases; neuropsychological problems; and other new directions for testing psychologists.

Facilities have been impacted by managed care to a marked degree. Cost containment and large cutbacks within various treatment venues are paradoxically countered by the ever-increasing performance expectations of patients, regulatory and accrediting bodies, and payors. Meeting these increased demands requires forward thinking as to the various economies afforded by expeditious testing methodologies, technologies, and protocols. Chapter 4 discusses a variety of models that offer cost savings while maintaining the goal of enhanced quality of clinical care.

Outcomes management is the focus of Chapter 5. The instrumentation and methodology considerations described include the psychologist's role in assessment of treatment outcome, treatment follow-up, patient satisfaction, and level of functioning. Chapter 6 reviews and explains various quality issues and reporting mechanisms such as the HEDIS Report Card, the JCAHO Report Card, the Baldrige National Quality Award standards developed for healthcare and other related areas, and how assessment can play a key role. Risk management, clinical liability, and the changing complexion of managing these areas within managed care cases are articulated in Chapter 7. Risks are increased and more complex within managed care. Various case precedents are provided, along with strategies for mitigating the risks.

Chapter 8 examines medical cost-offset issues, and provides statistics that are helpful in educating physicians, employers, and payors as to the merit, value, and cost savings afforded by application of psychological service to medical healthcare needs.

The book concludes with an in-depth look at automated systems for psychologists, who are now more mobile than they have been in the past. Telecommunications, accessibility, computer assistance, and cellular and other technologies help psychologists to provide better care and to manage their professional practice more efficiently. These technologies are continually improving even as they diminish in cost. This final chapter identifies some seeds from which enhancements and advancements may eventually grow.

I hope this book will be useful as psychologists adapt to changing circumstances. The goal is to provide various new ideas that will aid in attaining improved levels of clinical assessment and care while still maintaining high-quality practice standards and solidifying psychology's key role in healthcare.

CHRIS E. STOUT

Chicago, Illinois
January 1997

Contents

CONTENTS

SECTION IV

MANAGING TESTING SERVICES IN THE
NEW BEHAVIORAL FRONTIER

SECTION I

THE BRAVE NEW WORLD

CHAPTER 1

Where Managed Care Came From, and What It Means to Testing Psychologists

The Use of Psychological Tests

PSYCHOLOGICAL TESTING has long been an important and unique clinical application of psychology (Garfield, 1974; Goldenberg, 1973; Watson, 1953). The types and models of psychological assessment have not fundamentally changed over the past few decades (Sundberg, 1961; Watkins, Campbell, Nieberding, & Hallmark, 1995). The American Psychological Association's Clinical Division 12 (1993) views psychological testing activities as a key to defining clinical psychology. Piotrowski and his associates (Piotrowski & Keller, 1984; Piotrowski & Zalewiski, 1993) gathered strong evidence that psychological assessment, in its myriad forms, continues to be a prime component of graduate programs across the country. Watkins et al. (1995, p. 55) studied the contemporary private-practice activities of clinical psychologists and found:

- 90% conduct personality testing.
- 60% conduct intellectual assessment.
- 15% conduct vocational or career assessment.
- 13% conduct ability or aptitude testing.

Considering that the balance of their professional time must be spent on clinical psychology activities such as research, teaching, supervision, consultation, and administration, it is evident that personality

3

testing is second only to psychotherapy (96%) as an activity of practitioners. These findings apply across a variety of clinical settings—private practice, clinics, hospitals, and medical schools (Watkins et al., p. 58), and they highlight the importance and broad scope of psychological testing in clinical practice today.

The managed care reimbursement structures have had a marked impact on the prevalence of psychological testing. *Psychotherapy Finances,* a monthly newsletter devoted to practice aspects of behavioral healthcare providers, noted in a recent survey (Fee, Practice, and Managed Care Survey, 1995) that the number of psychologists who are providing testing services has now declined by approximately 10%. The decrease is likely amplified in an even greater decline in the testing evaluations conducted. This compounded result is of marked concern to psychology's role in behavioral healthcare.

Practice Impacts

Managed care has had a dramatic influence, both positive and negative, in the practice of behavioral healthcare. Clinicians, consultants, professional groups, and hospital administrators have argued against many managed care procedures. But, despite an initial dislike of managed care, it must be dealt with directly and proactively. Psychologists should work effectively within managed care for the best benefit of their patients while conducting their practice with the highest possible level of professionalism.

Managed Care's Evolution

HEALTH MAINTENANCE ORGANIZATIONS

Managed care, in its initial phases, was identified with health maintenance organizations (HMOs). This model provides enrollees with a variety of healthcare services, including behavioral healthcare, for a set payment amount per month. Often, HMOs are regulated by state insurance commissions. The most common practice models within HMOs are:

- *Staff Model*

  Clinicians are paid employees of the HMO.

  Care is provided at clinic sites that are owned and operated by the HMO.

- *Group Model*

  Clinicians are in a large private practice—or an Independent Practice Association (IPA) or Group Practice without Walls (GPWW)—that has broad geographic coverage through its various offices.

  Clinicians are *not* HMO employees (contrary to the Staff Model).

  Office sites are owned and operated by practice owners, not by the HMO.

  In some instances, a degree of exclusivity is provided to large group practices that receive the majority of referrals ("anchor groups").

- *Network Model*

  Similar to the Group Model, but uses a number of smaller practices to service clients, instead of a few large, anchor groups or IPAs/GPWWs.

FIRST GENERATION OF MANAGED CARE—SERVICE LIMITATIONS

The first generation of managed care consisted of rather unsophisticated service reduction. Payors paid for fewer days in inpatient and residential facilities. In addition, there was a limitation on the number of outpatient sessions. Psychological assessment was also limited. Frequently, psychological testing or assessment was simply not covered by a patient's insurance agreement. Along with service reduction, there was a reduction of the fees paid.

Psychologists' Payment Dilemmas

Testing psychologists found themselves in a variety of dilemmas with managed care cases. In some instances, regardless of what test was administered in the battery, they would be paid a flat fee. However, some managed care companies would pay for only certain types of tests; other companies would not pay at all. If a utilization reviewer or case manager felt that psychological testing was not indicated (even if testing was a covered benefit), then testing would not be approved, even after it had been ordered by the doctor in charge of the case. A variety of payment schemes have been effected, other than limiting the amount paid for a full battery or for select tests. Psychological testing within the managed care environment is sometimes paid for, at a reduced hourly rate, for an unlimited number of hours.

Payment Examples

The most frequent methods of pricing and payment are:

- *Flat Rate* (or *Fee for Battery*). A testing battery is paid for, if approved within a policy's benefit structure, at a total set fee, regardless of the number and types of tests administered or the amount of time taken. There is usually an implicit (if not explicit) minimum expectation of an intelligence test, an objective personality measure, and an interview or screening device or two. Fee rates may range from $250 to $500, depending on the payor, the geographic region, and the minimal tests included.
- *Fee-for-Test.* Reimbursement is based on a predetermined selection of approved tests at approved fees. Usually, there is no option to bill for the additional time involved in interpretation or in writing the report. Thus, if an examiner wishes to administer the Wexler Adult Intelligence Test-Revised (WAIS-R) and Minnesota Multiphasic Personality Inventory-Second Edition (MMPI-2), and conduct a clinical interview (presuming all are approved), payment would be based on the total of the sum of each test's predetermined reimbursement level. Thus, if the managed care organization reimburses

$75.00 for WAIS-R, $50.00 for MMPI-2, and $100.00 for a clinical interview, the battery would yield $225.00.

- *Fee-for-Service.* Reimbursement is based on an hourly rate. For example, if 5 hours are billed for administration and scoring, the 5 hours are multiplied by the customary managed care rate for testing (usually, $70 per hour) to yield the total fee allowed (i.e., $350).

   Some plans may limit the total hours per battery (or per testing episode), even though testing may take longer. Other plans may not limit hours but may require preapproval and may possibly dictate which tests to be administered. (The preapproval process of the flat rate is similar; see below.)

   More generous plans may pay for the time it takes to write the report. Examiners must be aware of a possible requirement for using different Current Procedural Terminology (CPT) coding in such instances (e.g., CPT 90887: Results Interpretation, or CPT 90889: Preparation of Report). When examiners bill for their services, it is very important to use the appropriate CPT code to avoid any risk of nonpayment or any question of insurance fraud. (Such risks are discussed in detail in Chapter 7.)

- *Inclusive/Per Diem/Capitated Rate.* Arrangements with facilities, group practices, or other types of provider entities may contract for a variety of services "bundled" together. If psychological testing is part of that bundle, it is unlikely that any "independent contractor" examiner would be referred to the case. These arrangements typically occur within hospitals or other systems of care. A staff psychologist who is on salary (or retainer, or some other similar employment arrangement) conducts the referred testing and bills no one. There is usually no preapproval or regulation/restriction as to test selection or battery composition. Such choices are within the discretion and clinical judgment of the assessor.

Summaries of Payment Models

Table 1.1 offers a comparative analysis of the various reimbursement models for psychological assessment under the current managed care options.

TABLE 1.1

A Sample Comparison of "Standard" Testing Battery Reimbursement Models

Battery Components	Flat Rate Test/Activities Included		Fee for Test Test/Activities Included		Fee for Service* Test/Activities Included		Capitated Test/Activities Included	
	Yes	Amount	Yes	Amount	Yes	Amount	Yes	Amount
Clinical interview	✓	N/A	✓	$ 75	✓	$ 70	✓	$0
Bender gestalt	✓	N/A			✓	20	✓	0
WAIS-R	✓	N/A	✓	75	✓	100	✓	0
MMPI-2	✓	N/A	✓	50	✓	50	✓	0
TAT	✓	N/A			✓	50	✓	0
Rorschach	✓	N/A					✓	0
Aphasia screen	✓	N/A			✓	25	✓	0
Score/Interpretation	✓	N/A					✓	0
Report write-up	✓	N/A					✓	0
Total paid		$300		$225		$315		$0**

* Amount based on fraction of $70/hour.

** Psychologist is paid per member, per month (PMPM), not per discrete clinical activity.

Concerns Involving Payment Decision Makers

This author attended a managed care conference in which a psychiatrist, who was a medical director of a managed care company, stated, "The day that I see a scientific research study that indicates that the Rorschach is a valid and a reliable tool for assessing an individual's level of psychopathology is the day that I will pay for one." This statement highlights several unreconciled issues:

1. Individuals without training in psychological testing, psychometric procedures, or statistical analysis may make determinations as to what type of testing is or is not appropriate.
2. There is definitely a consistent bias within the managed care industry toward objective tests and away from projective types of tests.
3. Broadly, psychology needs to demonstrate (from both psychometric and fiscal perspectives) the merit of such assessment in improving the quality of care and clinical efficiency, and adding cost-effective value. More specifically, it is incumbent on testing psychologists to structure a test battery that best

fits referral needs while still operating within the guidelines of *each* managed care company's contract.

SECOND GENERATION OF MANAGED CARE—PREFERRED PROVIDER ORGANIZATIONS

The preferred provider organization (PPO) is the second generation of managed care. In this model, select providers contract for provision of specific types of services at preset, reduced fees. The patient has the option to use an independent provider, but there are financial disincentives for going outside the payor/insurance network—for example, a higher co-pay or deductible, or less reimbursement for that clinician. At present, there is no federal level of regulation for PPOs.

Utilization Review and Management

The additional component of second-generation managed care is the initiation of utilization review/utilization management (UR/UM). Staff are responsible for interfacing with facilities or providers in approving treatment plans or procedures such as psychological testing. Historically, there has been a great deal of friction and frustration between clinicians and utilization review managers. Initially, some utilization reviewers of managed care companies were not clinically trained. Fortunately, as things have evolved, individuals in these positions have become more sophisticated, and managed care companies increasingly use psychiatric nurses, psychiatrists, psychologists, and professionals in this capacity. Thus, UR/UM is now a peer-to-peer model. (Chapter 7 examines a case precedent regarding the legal history of clinical responsibility of care, regardless of payor or facility support.)

Application Expectations

Applications of PPOs are not standardized, which can create a confusing array of paperwork for clinicians attempting to join the organizations. However, most managed care organizations (MCOs) do require the following documents:

1. Proof of malpractice insurance (usually a copy of the face sheet and amounts in the range of $1 million per occurrence/$1 million per annual aggregate, or $1 million per occurrence/$3 million per annual aggregate).
2. Copy of professional license.
3. Copy of diploma of terminal degree.
4. One to three letters of recommendation.
5. Copy of National Practitioner Databank Query results (800-767-6732 or 805-987-9476).
6. Documentation of any malpractice history.
7. Sample report and/or treatment plan.
8. Description of treatment or clinical philosophy.
9. Current vita.
10. The MCO's own application.

Many psychologists will find it helpful to keep copies of these documents on hand in order to expedite processing applications. The American Managed Behavioral Healthcare Association (AMBHA), which has the country's largest managed behavioral healthcare firms as members, is working on the development of a standardized application and uniform credentials requirements.

THIRD GENERATION OF MANAGED CARE—
AUTOMATION AND MANAGED CARE

The third generation of managed care involves a greater number of automated systems. There has been rapid improvement in the sophistication and utilization of these systems. Managed Health Network uses a very innovative combination of "bubble" forms and bar coding to expeditiously process claims. CNR and US Behavioral Health have contracted with InStream™—a data processing company partnered with AT&T™—for an innovative, on-site data entry system that is being used throughout the United States. A variety of different utilization tracking methodologies are being employed; some of the more sophisticated methods use provider profiling, diagnosis cross-validation, and computer-administered therapy.

FOURTH GENERATION OF MANAGED CARE— OUTCOMES MANAGEMENT

The fourth generation is considered to be the advent of outcomes, with a focus on efficacy and outcomes management systems. (Outcomes management systems are discussed in Chapter 5.) Outcomes management includes evaluation and quantified measurement of patient satisfaction, symptom resolution (treatment outcome), functionality measures, and demonstrated efficacy (outcome follow-up). The increasing focus on outcomes makes quality a more robust part of the managed care equation. This is operationalized by the examination of clinical performance data in relation to clinical procedures. Psychological assessment in its various forms (e.g., screening tools, specific instruments, health status measures, batteries, and so on) can play a strong role in this iteration of managed care. However, it is psychologists' responsibility to champion this integration. They should not wait for the managed care industry to do so.

FIFTH GENERATION OF MANAGED CARE—CAPITATION AND RISK SHARING

The fifth generation of managed care is considered by most of the industry to be capitation and risk sharing. Service delivery utilizes a prenegotiated, fixed payment (or premium) that is prepaid on a per member, per month (PMPM) basis to the provider/facility, for which enrollees receive a predetermined set of services for a contracted time period. The fee must be paid regardless of services provided. Psychological testing is unlikely to be a "carved-out" (i.e., not included) component within a capitated arrangement. Thus, it is very important for psychologists whose practices are solely focused on testing to become part of a group practice (or a number of group practices or facilities) as subcontractors for testing services. The prediction is that most managed care arrangements will shift to capitation within the next two to five years.

A variety of books and other publications discuss managing capitation and contracts and how to develop PMPM rates. Such information in any further detail is beyond the scope of this book. However, interested readers may contact Business Network (800-889-2688) or the Institute for Behavioral Healthcare (415-435-7820) for books, tapes, and seminar schedules.

GENERATIONAL OVERLAP

In this evolutionary model, there are no discrete steps of progression. Quite the contrary occurs in the healthcare marketplace: most of the five evolutions coexist simultaneously, with ever-changing proportions of penetration. Differences are found in various geographic regions. California tends to be the trendsetter that the country follows for managed behavioral healthcare reimbursement models.

Managed Care's Impact on Psychology

The Practice Directorate of the American Psychological Association recently commissioned a focus group research project (APAPD, 1994) on managed care using the Widmeyer Group, Inc. The project was conducted in four cities with six focus groups. The findings indicated a consensus among those surveyed. The primary findings noted in the report (p. 1) are as follows:

1. *"Eroding Self-Confidence."* This erosion was identified less with the profession of psychology than with its position within the economic scheme of healthcare.
2. *"Loss of Control."* Psychologists perceived threats to their identity as healthcare providers and to their ability to function and practice independently.
3. *"Feeling Vulnerable."* Economic erosion within the practice of psychology was being experienced by those surveyed. Concerns included public perceptions and misperceptions of how psychologists practice.
4. *"Disturbed by Trends."* Some psychologists are considering leaving the field in response to unforeseen changes and shifts

within their psychological practice in particular, and health-care delivery in general. Actual feelings of loss and mourning were noted with regard to these changes.

The APAPD study also explored respondents' direct opinions concerning managed care. The psychologists polled felt that (p. 2):

1. *"Providing quality or preventive care is not enough of a priority for managed care."* Psychologists pointed to what they felt was a lack of treatment quality within managed care plans. Cost containment was a greater worry than quality, and the medical model was a poor fit to psychological problems and treatments.
2. *"Continuing erosion of the right to confidentiality."* Ethical and legal issues are involved when patients' reports and other clinical data are discussed with a utilization reviewer. The expertise and training of reviewers were a related issue.
3. *"Managed care raises serious ethical issues."* Problems with appropriate utilization of diagnostic codes were described, as was the perceived balancing act of not-too-sick-but-not-too-well as a contrived means of keeping a patient in care (i.e., improvement and lack of improvement are *both* causes for a treatment's termination).
4. *"Managed care makes everyone do more for less."* This concern alludes to psychologists' perception that treatment expectations are waxing while concomitant payment levels are waning.
5. *"The person reviewing cases does not understand psychologists' work."* This response is parallel to the above-noted concern about the credentials of utilization reviewers. Problems herein seem to result from reviews that are not peer-to-peer.

MARKET-DRIVEN FORCES WITHIN PSYCHOLOGICAL PRACTICE

Notwithstanding the earlier description of the generations of managed care, the practitioner may not understand the driving forces behind these impacts, the currently changing complexion of health-care, and the possibilities that national healthcare reform may hold. Drum (1995), in an excellent overview and summary, sees seven forces as being responsible for the changes that psychologists are currently facing.

1. "Traditional" third-party indemnity health insurance policies simply passed on increases in providers' cost (i.e., fees charged) to the second-party employers. In this way, the profit margins of third-party insurers could remain stable (or linearly increase) over time from a minimal to a moderate rate. Morrison (personal communication, July 6, 1995) argues that there was no utilization control because of the lack of third-party payors' accountability. Instead of psychological testing serving as a driving force when making referrals and triage, it was often just added on as a profit center. Drum notes that, over time, such pass-through increases became less easy for the second-party employers to absorb. New ways to maintain profit margins had to be found. Providers were then targeted via the application of cost containment measures, as noted previously in first generation managed care: fewer services at lower reimbursement levels.

2. Psychologists fought diligently in the 1970s to gain reimbursement, through insurance policies, for most clinical services. Various states, as a result of psychologists' vigorous political efforts, adopted freedom of choice laws, which led to a dependence by many licensed psychologists on insurance reimbursement as a key source of income. Drum indicates that this has additionally caused many psychologists to build their practice around such reimbursement structures. Now that this model is in flux and change, it becomes incumbent on psychologists to adapt to new developments and paradigms.

3. Traditional economic tenets of supply-and-demand effects on pricing and costs did not seem applicable to the oversupply of providers (e.g., psychologists, psychiatrists, social workers, and counselors) versus the number of people in need of behavioral healthcare services (Drum, 1995). This also contributed to the ever-increasing costs associated with behavioral healthcare, the insurers' need to increase cost control measures, and fertile ground for new managed care concepts.

14

4. Drum's fourth point concerns an almost phenomenological "discovery by corporate America that the healthcare industry can be organized into a competitive market" (p. 5).

5. Next came the epiphenomenon of cost shifting from the dollars saved via reduced payments to providers and facilities. These savings (with the exception of copayments) are afforded to patients and employers, and profits to insurers and managed care organizations are increased.

6. Aggressive Darwinian forces of market share have driven healthcare corporations toward economic dominance. For providers, this operationally translates into more technical expectations (e.g., utilization reviews, increased paperwork, outcome and satisfaction studies, and so on) while getting paid less for the actual clinical services rendered and the additional stress of increased "clinical competition" via restrictive or limited network application acceptance (e.g., PPOs becoming "closed").

7. At the federal level, the two major political parties have politicized healthcare in the government's failed attempt at reform. The cost increases experienced by business are mimicked in the parallel increase in federal spending on healthcare and the finite inability to raise taxes as much as would be necessary to continue to fund such care. Psychologists are continually caught in these issues.

PRACTICE PREDICTIONS

Cummings (1985, 1986, 1992) has long championed the idea that health maintenance organizations and other non-indemnity-based care and payment systems are harbingers of the future. His current (1995) perspective continues with a hopeful view for the delivery of psychological services. He predicts that "behavioral healthcare carveouts will disappear" (p. 31). They will simply no longer be necessary, as a result of technical advances and of buyers' and employers' better understanding of psychology's weaknesses and benefits. Cummings sees this as a necessary evolutionary step in the continuing industrialization of healthcare and psychological practice.

15

Cummings' second prediction (1995, p. 31) is that "medical cost offset will become the most regarded outcomes research." The literature is replete with research demonstrating the efficacy of psychological care in decreasing subsequent (and more expensive) biological healthcare needs and costs. (This is noted in greater detail in Chapter 8.) The third prediction suggests that master's-level "technicians" will conduct psychotherapy, and doctoral-level psychologists will focus more on the administrative, supervisory, and evaluative aspects of care. A greater reliance on outcomes-supported care will drive this system of the future. Psychometricians, and similarly trained non-doctoral-level psychologists, may be the clinicians conducting psychological testing.

"Community consortia will emerge and dictate the market" is Cummings's (1995, p. 31) fourth prediction. The "consortia" are the purchasers of care who design quality and breadth of psychological services as well as cost savings. His final prediction suggests that "the delivery systems of the future will be the community accountable healthcare networks (CAHNs)" (p. 31). These networks are basically coordinated continua of care: integrated inpatient, outpatient, partial hospitalization/day treatment, residential, aftercare, in-home, and other newly developed venues of treatment. Psychological testing, as well as psychotherapy, will be provided. This type of system will be ideally positioned to manage fully capitated and shared-risk contracts. Psychologist-hospital organizations (PHOs) are likely to play a role in some of these structures as well as in other new ventures and buyouts.

CLINICAL PRACTICE CHANGES IN MANAGED CARE

To be best prepared for various managed care circumstances, psychologists need to be conversant with typical case management expectations. Anderson and Berlant (1994) note four overlapping key factors:

1. **The need for correct diagnosis and effective treatment.** This author (Stout, 1989, 1990) has long noted that accurate diagnosis is the sine qua non of appropriate treatment planning and maximal outcome and prognosis. Additionally, misdiagnosis may lead to various liability risks: failure

16

to accurately diagnose, failure to adequately treat, and perhaps failure to refer (Stout, 1994; VandeCreek & Stout, 1993). From this perspective, psychological testing's role may be a key component to improving diagnostic accuracy and certainty, resulting in improved treatment planning and care, while managing and mitigating clinical liability risk.

2. **The case manager's function of fostering the most "efficient use of resources."** Anderson and Berlant (1994) differentiate utilization review as striving "to exclude payment for unnecessarily intensive treatment, whereas case management strives to direct patients into effective forms of treatment at appropriate levels of intensity" (p. 135). This difference is fundamental and marked; however, many practicing psychologists do not yet understand such differences and often view utilization review as analogous to case management.

3. **Decreasing costly procedures.** Episodic, acute contacts over time may be totally appropriate with some insurance plans and policies.

4. **Avoiding poor quality services.** The application of quality improvement principles to behavioral healthcare is gaining considerable interest, support, and momentum. This is excellent for both clinical practice and resultant patient care. (More discussion of this topic is in Chapter 6.)

NEGATIVE PRACTICE IMPACTS

With the possible exception of some capitated, shared-risk contracts, psychologists must realize that being in a preferred provider network may result in a decrease of revenues. On average, approximately 10% to 35% less per service (depending on the market) will be realized. Psychologists who specialize in assessment may experience an additional 10% to 25% decrease in annual revenues if their practices and payor mix (their various payor sources—Medicare, indemnity, private payment, managed care, and so on) had previously not been markedly penetrated by managed care as a result of denials for testing. As noted in the discussion of the first generation of managed

17

care, annual practice income is usually diminished by two factors: (a) a decrease in usual and customary per-procedure fees, and (b) a decrease in clinical activities (i.e., as with therapy sessions, this decrease is represented in testing limitations or denials of assessment).

PRACTICE GROWTH WITHIN MANAGED CARE, AND CONTRACT ISSUES

More sophisticated MCOs are now moving toward requesting providers to identify the volume of patients seen, according to their zip code, diagnostic group, age group, patient satisfaction, and various outcome measures, and to list their own continuing education credits. In this author's opinion, the sophistication of data required for credentialing and recredentialing will increase significantly in the near future. Once an application is approved, a provider agreement or a contract is typically sent to the clinician. Such a contract should be read in detail, taken very seriously, and reviewed by the clinician's legal counsel prior to signing. It is incumbent on the clinician to be certain that the contract's requirements and obligations are clearly understood. Stout, Theis, and Oher's (1996) guidebook on managed care discusses in detail what to expect in various contracts. Some MCOs have rather unexpected clauses, such as a "no complaining to patients" agreement that actually prohibits contracted providers from saying to a patient something perceived as negative about the MCO. It is quite worthwhile to seriously examine any and all contracts as a standard office/practice procedure and policy.

Practice Operation Tips

In contracting with managed care companies, testing psychologists will likely be asked about the following practice components. All psychologists are well advised to consider designing their practice to adequately meet these issues:

1. Geographic areas that can be serviced.
2. Medical/Professional staff membership status at local hospitals or medical centers.

3. Facility for prompt return of phone calls.
4. Appointment availability.
5. New referral capacity/limitations.
6. Number of networks/PPOs/HMOs in which the psychologist is currently a provider.
7. Sample reports for various diagnostic categories and populations.
8. Testing/treatment "philosophy" or orientation.
9. Liability history and outcomes.
10. Fee structure by:

    - CPT Code.
    - Procedure/test.
    - Battery type (e.g., psychological; neuropsychological; developmental; intellectual).

11. Level of automation (e.g., computer, Electronic Data Interchange (EDI), fax, Internet, voice mail, etc.).

Psychologists may find it very useful to develop a list or even a matrix of the managed care and insurance companies they belong to, and to list, for each one, the criteria, contracts, phone numbers, and so on, for precertifications, payment types (e.g., FFS, FFT, Flat Rate, etc.), payment levels, and other relevant data. Frequent reference to this list will ensure that any and all procedural needs to conduct testing and to avoid denial of payment for services rendered have been met. A sample matrix appears in Figure 1.1.

Additional Opportunities

Although this book focuses on various healthcare settings and managed care, it is important to note that testing psychologists may find opportunities to provide services in additional areas. The examples provided below are not exhaustive; they are intended to stimulate thought and consideration. Many areas are not, and perhaps will not be, impacted by managed care regulations. Ethically,

Managed Care Organization/ Insurance Company	Testing Pre-certification Required?	Contact Person (Discipline)	Position	Phone Number	Fax Number	Billing Address	Payment Type	Payment Level	Additional Information
XYZ Corp.	Yes	Dr. Jones (Psychologist)	Utilization Reviewer	800-555-8900	800-555-8901	111 Anywhere Dr. Your Town, USA	Flat Rate	$350/battery	Rapid payment, w/in 30 days
ABC Group	No	Ms. Smith (Social Worker)	Utilization Reviewer	800-555-1111	800-555-1112	222 Backstreet My Town, USA	FFS	$70/hour	Max of 5 hrs/battery include write-up

FIGURE 1.1
Managed Care Matrix

whatever type of service is provided, the testing psychologist must be adequately trained in all procedural factors prior to providing the service.

The suggested additional service categories are:

1. Industrial/Occupational:

   Employee selection.

   Employee advancement.

   Employee suitability (e.g., overseas transfer-candidate selection).

   Employee job matching.

   Workers' compensation issues.

   Specialist candidate evaluations:

   - Police officer.
   - Firefighter.
   - Nuclear plant hiree.

2. Forensic:

   "Not guilty by reason of insanity" cases.

   Competency to stand trial.

   General competency hearings.

   Child custody cases.

   Workers' compensation adjudication.

   Expert witness testing/testimony.

   Juror selection.

3. Educational/Academic: Child

   Learning disabilities.

   Behavioral disorders.

   Emotional disorders.

   ADHD/ADD.

   IDEA (P.L. 101-476) and Section 504 (Rehabilitation Act) issues.

4. Educational/Academic: Adult

   Independent evaluations.

   Due process hearings.

   Learning disabilities evaluations.

   Americans with Disabilities Act evaluations (e.g., employ-ment/environment adaptations to a learning disability).

Conclusion

With all of the challenges facing testing psychologists today, it is important to consider taking the strong, proactive steps noted herein for practice survival. No book or plan can guarantee success, but the methods and ideas noted throughout this volume are intended to serve as a helpful guide.

SECTION II

THE GOOD NEWS:
NEW ARENAS FOR
PSYCHOLOGICAL ASSESSMENT

CHAPTER 2

Psychological Assessment in Primary Care Settings

W ITH THE ADVENT OF health maintenance organizations (HMOs), primary care physicians have had the additional role of "gatekeeper" thrust upon them. The intent with this model is to have a centralized medical generalist serve as the initial contact for patients, regardless of their presenting complaint(s) or symptoms. Many HMOs and some managed care companies utilize this model instead of a direct referral to a behavioral healthcare provider. Anderson and Berlant (1994) note that, in some models of managed care, the primary care physician (PCP) will actually provide psychiatric diagnoses and clinical care in more straightforward cases.

Diagnostic Problems of Primary Care Physicians

From a management utilization perspective, the favorable aspects of having PCPs provide screening/assessment, triage, referral, and/or treatment are self-evident. Anderson and Berlant (1994) point out the benefits of centralized clinical authority and continuity of care. Phenomenologically, it is not surprising that many individuals with vague somatic complaints may initially present to a physician instead of a psychologist. However, the key disadvantage of having PCPs act as behavioral healthcare gatekeepers is that they tend to be poor behavioral diagnosticians (Wells, Stewart, Hays, et al., 1989). Fifer (1994) found that primary care physicians working in HMO settings frequently underdiagnosed present anxiety, and thus did not effectively treat or refer patients who had clinical levels of anxiety. Fifer concluded that such diagnostic errors of omission result from a lack of reliable medical profiles, demographic characteristics, or premorbid traits that act as cues within the practice of most primary care physicians. It is important to build strong, comprehensive practice ties between testing psychologists and these physicians.

Kelleher (1995) notes the concern with PCPs' poor psychodiagnostic abilities. "Unrecognized mental disorder diagnoses account for between 30% and 80% of all cases seen in primary care settings. . . . Primary care clinicians (themselves) report that they have too little training, time, or confidence in mental health services to more effectively treat patients with mental disorders" (pp. 1, 3). PCPs also noted dissatisfaction with the *Diagnostic and Statistical Manual of Mental Disorders*, Third Edition, Revised (DSM-III-R), because, from their perspective, their specialty received meager offerings of the symptom complexes to which PCPs are accustomed (Kelleher, 1995).

Tools to Aid Primary Care Physicians

DSM-IV-PC

Members of the behavioral healthcare community have made a number of attempts to address the issues posed by having PCPs serve as gatekeepers in the behavioral health arena. These disadvantages have been targeted by various groups as an area in which to provide diagnostic assistance. For example, the American Psychiatric Association has just published its first manual on psychiatric and substance abuse disorders written for primary care physicians (Baldwin, 1995a). With the words *Primary Care* appended to the title, it is basically a revised edition of the American Psychiatric Association's *Diagnostic and Statistical Manual of Mental Disorders*, Fourth Edition, and is identified as DSM-IV-PC. It took over four years to produce and incorporate considerations from the specialties of family medicine, internal medicine, obstetrics, gynecology, and pediatrics. This new symptom-driven manual leads users through various clinical decision possibilities that would indicate the likely presence of the more common psychiatric disorders that may manifest and first present to PCPs. These include: depression, sleep problems, sexual disturbances, anxiety, and other unexplained general physical complaints (Baldwin, 1995a).

PRIME-MD

Pfizer, Inc., a pharmaceutical manufacturer, has sponsored the development, by the New York State Psychiatric Institute's Biometrics Research Department, of a diagnostic instrument intended to aid PCPs in identifying anxiety, depression, eating disorders, and substance abuse disorders. The result is a patient questionnaire entitled PRIME-MD (Primary Care Evaluation of Mental Disorders). Baldwin (1995b) notes the PRIME-MD is composed of two sections. The first is a 26-item yes-or-no survey concerning a patient's experiences with various psychiatric signs and symptoms within the past month. It is designed to be self-administered prior to the physician visit. The second component is a 12-page clinical evaluation guide (CEG) that serves as a structured interview for the physician's follow-up to affirmative symptom responses by the patient on the self-administered survey. The CEG's goal is to streamline further data collection of flagged areas of patient distress (e.g., stomach, back, or chest pain; sleep disturbance; fatigue; gastrointestinal distress; depressed feelings; worry; alcohol consumption levels; or eating problems).

A recent study (Spitzer et al., 1994b), conducted by the questionnaire's authors and sponsored by Pfizer, found PRIME-MD helpful in identifying 26% of the 1,000 patient subjects tested as meeting full criteria for a specific disorder in the DSM-III-R. The study indicated that it took 8.4 minutes for the average PCP to complete a PRIME-MD evaluation, and an overall accuracy rate of 88% was achieved. This is particularly important in light of a finding that PCPs typically fail to diagnose between 50% and 75% of patients who present for medical care when indeed they are in need of behavioral healthcare intervention (Eastman, 1995). A free copy of the questionnaire is available from:

PRIME-MD
c/o Pfizer, Inc.
235 E. 42nd Street
New York, NY 10017-5755

SDDS-PC

Using a similar approach, the Upjohn Company has developed the Symptom-Driven Diagnosis System—Primary Care (SDDS-PC), an automated two-step diagnostic screening device for psychopathology. Like PRIME-MD, the SDDS-PC is designed for use by primary care physicians, from early identification and triage to treatment or further diagnostic evaluation. The SDDS-PC's first component is a patient self-administered form. Subsequently, the physician administers additional diagnostic modules. The physician also receives forms for longitudinal tracking of cases. SDDS-PC is available from:

The Upjohn Company
7000 Portage Road
Kalamazoo, MI 49001

Select Psychological Instruments

MBHI

The DSM-IV-PC, PRIME-MD, and SDDS-PC are intended specifically for use by primary care physicians. Among other instruments designed to tap into psychological issues relevant to medical patients is the Millon Behavioral Health Inventory (MBHI), which examines a patient's psychological coping styles and how they may impact medical care. The following scales comprise the MBHI:

Basic Coping Styles	Psychogenic Attitudes	Psychosomatic Correlates	Prognostic Indicators
Introversive	Chronic Tension	Allergic Inclination	Pain Treatment Responsibility
Inhibited	Relevant Stress	Gastrointestinal Susceptibility	Life Threat Reactivity
Cooperative	Premorbid Pessimism	Cardiovascular Tendency	Emotional Vulnerability
Sociable	Future Despair		
Confident	Social Alienation		
Forceful	Somatic Anxiety		
Respectful			
Sensitive			

The MBHI is a self-administered inventory of 150 true/false items. It requires an eighth-grade reading level and approximately 20 minutes to complete. It is limited to adult patients and is available in paper-and-pencil, online, and audiocassette versions, in English or Spanish. Medical applications include (NCS, 1995, p. 53):

1. Evaluation/screening of physically ill, injured, and surgical patients to help identify possible psychosomatic complications or predict response to illness or treatment.
2. Workers' compensation evaluations to help assess stress-related claims and establish rehabilitation programs.
3. Evaluation/screening of individuals in specialty clinics or programs (e.g., for pain, stress, or headache) who have a psychological disorder or an unidentified stressor.

16PF

The Sixteen Personality Factor (16PF) instrument, devised by Cattell, is used in a wide variety of clinical, vocational, and academic settings. With medical patients, 16PF is used to assist in clinical diagnosis, prognosis, psychotherapeutic treatment planning, and differential medication selection.

The instrument is a 187-item self-report questionnaire that is applicable to patients 16 years of age or older, who have at least a seventh-grade reading level. Approximately 45 to 60 minutes are needed to complete it in a paper-and-pencil or online version. It provides information on 16 continua of personality dimensions (NCS, 1995, p. 96).

MMPI-2

The Minnesota Multiphasic Personality Inventory-2 (MMPI-2) is a classic objective test of adult psychopathology. Many of its scales are applicable with medical patients, such as hypochondriasis (Scale 1, Hs) and conversion hysteria (Scale 3, Hy). Testing psychologists are likely to be very conversant with MMPI and MMPI-2. However, the additional scales listed in Table 2.1 offer rich information that is applicable to medical populations (NCS, 1995, p. 7).

P-3

The Post-Traumatic Personality Profile (P-3) is a relatively new, brief tool that is self-administered and provides information dealing with psychological factors (e.g., depression, anxiety, and somatization) associated with pain. Tollison and Langley (NCS, 1995, p. 65) designed the P-3 for assessing pain resulting from traumatic events such as accidents, but it is also appropriate for cancer, arthritis, and other biologically caused types of pain. P-3 is for adults with a minimum sixth-grade reading level and consists of 48 multiple-choice statements. Paper-and-pencil administration takes about 15 to 20 minutes.

LEVEL-OF-FUNCTIONING MEASURES

Assessment of level of functioning is gaining increasing attention within managed care payor systems. The phrase *level of functioning*

TABLE 2.1
MMPI-2: Additional Scales Relevant to Medical Populations

Clinical Scales	Supplementary Scales
(1) Hs Hypochondriasis	MAC-R MacAndrew Alcoholism-
(3) Hy Conversion Hysteria	Revised

Content Scales	*Harris-Lingoes Subscales*
HEA Health Concerns	D_2 Psychomotor Retardation
TPA Type A	D_3 Physical Malfunctioning
	Hy_3 Lassitude-Malaise
Content Component Scales	Hy_4 Somatic Complaints
Depression Subscales	**Setting-Specific Indexes**
DEP4 Suicidal Ideation	Pain Classification

Health Concerns Subscales

HEA1   Gastrointestinal Symptoms
HEA2   Neurological Symptoms
HEA3   General Health Concerns

Negative Treatment Indicators
TRT1   Low Motivation
TRT2   Inability to Disclose

can have a variety of meanings to those using the term. For some, it is simply a patient's Axis V ranking within DSM-III-R or DSM-IV. For others, it may mean health or medical functional status; or, it may refer to pragmatic lifestyle issues such as returning to work, staying sober or drug-free, staying out of jail, and so forth. As time passes, this area will surely develop and advance, acquiring a clearer consensus as to how it will be conceptualized, defined, quantified, and monitored. Listings of some of the functional measurement instruments now in use appear in the Appendix. Additional information concerning functional measures is given in Chapter 5.

Psychology's Impact

In terms of strategic positioning, it is important for testing psychologists to educate primary care physicians, pediatricians, internists, and other medical generalists and specialists as to the beneficial aspects of referral for in-depth psychological testing. Psychologists must be sensitive to:

1. Costs of testing.
2. Whether the referring physician may "lose" the patient (i.e., a testing referral may lead to a therapy referral that could result in the patient's leaving the referring physician's practice in order to be seen by a specialist).
3. Whether testing provides an "added value" for the patient or the referring physician.

Additional considerations that may aid psychologists in promoting testing referrals via the development of a strong marketing plan and related materials are discussed in detail in Chapter 8.

REFERRAL RECOMMENDATIONS

Correct referral and treatment recommendations are extremely important for testing psychologists working for PCPs. Psychologists need to be aware of the clinical interventions that may be appropriate for patients with medical illnesses. Shumaker (1990) notes various types of psychological interventions associated with biological disorders. For example, a cancer patient who has lost a limb or is experiencing loss of hair via chemotherapy would require additional symptom-related interventions (e.g., psychotherapy to deal with issues of self-esteem, embarrassment, adaptation to hair loss, and changed appearance). Non-symptom-related interventions would involve the more traditional psychological concerns associated with the stresses and problems of coping with a major illness (e.g., depression, anger, guilt, anxiety). Diagnosis-related interventions would be recommended after psychological evaluation concerning emotional functioning in relation to pre- or postoperative status. Additional interventions and considerations include (Shumaker, 1990, p. 142):

Intervention	Consideration
Diagnostic	Neuropsychological functioning concerns
	Pre-/postoperative psychological evaluation
	Differential diagnosis
	General psychological functioning
Symptom-related	Adjustment to:
	Acute/chronic illness or condition
	Surgical procedure
	Trauma
	General concerns with diagnosed medical problem(s)
	Compliance with prescribed medical regimes
Non-symptom-related	Dysfunction in:
	Interpersonal relationship(s)
	Employment
	Life adjustment
	Affective disorders
	Stressors not related to a diagnosed medical disorder

Psychological Practice Expansion with Medical Patients: Improving Quality While Decreasing Costs

Cummings and Follette (1968; Follette & Cummings, 1967) noted three decades ago that psychiatric patients with physical illnesses may experience an exacerbation of both their psychological and their medical problems. When such individuals present to physicians not trained in psychiatry, the likelihood of misdiagnosis of the medical problem is heightened, as is the likelihood of nondiagnosis of the psychiatric disorder. Thus, testing psychologists may consider offering their consultative services to general medical/surgical hospitals. Strumwasser et al. (1991) suggest that if such testing occurred at preadmission, a 30% reduction in unnecessary psychiatric patient admissions and a 60% reduction in substance abuse patient admissions might be realized. Such a procedure, modified to site-specific needs, policies, and procedures, would be relevant within managed care arrangements and of particular importance to facilities that host capitated, shared-risk plans. The need for such innovations is heightened by the growing focus on improving quality of patient care.

Walen (1985) discovered that medical patients with a co-morbid psychological diagnosis tend to have longer overall lengths of stay (10.8 days) as compared to matched cohorts who do not have the psychological diagnosis (7.3 days). Fulop, Strain, Hammer, and Lyons (1989) investigated two hospitals in large metropolitan cities and found that psychiatrically and medically diagnosed inpatients had up to double the length of stay compared to those who had only a medical diagnosis. Investigators (Lyons, Hammer, Strain, & Fulop, 1986; Mumford, Schlesinger, & Glass, 1982) found that one or two fewer days of hospitalization were necessary when these patients were provided with psychotherapeutic services. Within a more specific methodological examination, Fulop, Strain, Hammer, and Lyons (1989, January) found that *certain* medical diagnostic categories were exacerbated by co-morbid psychiatric diagnoses. These include (p. 81):

1. Neoplasms.
2. Circulatory disorders.
3. Digestive disorders.
4. Renal disorders.
5. Respiratory disorders.

Physicians treating patients with problems in these areas should strongly consider psychological evaluation and the possibility of psychotherapeutic services. Managed care organizations would also need to become more aware of such enhancements to overall quality patient care while simultaneously decreasing the costs associated with extended inpatient lengths of stay.

Psychologists must keep in mind that many physicians are not familiar with the value and aid of psychological testing. They are, however, familiar with the need for lab tests and the merits of collegial consultations. Thus, it is helpful to train physicians to conceptualize psychological tests as being similar to lab tests—consultative tools to aid in problem discovery, symptom understanding, diagnostic formulation, and treatment planning. When physicians learn the value of such testing, they tend to utilize it more.

The Importance of Psychological Testing in HMOs

Medical patients in HMOs are unlikely to consistently visit the same physician. Economies afforded by interchangeable, equally skilled technician-physicians are now the norm. This practicality of contemporary medical practice in tandem with typically episodic contact can result in a physician's not having a full historical understanding or conceptualization of the patient. The prognostic accuracy of the physician is then impeded (Eber, 1977). Personality traits, lifestyle choices, habits, and other psychological variables play a multicausal role in illness development and health risks. Brief, episodic, and (physical) symptom-focused contacts do not provide physicians with the data necessary to conceptualize a patient's general level of functioning (Eber, 1977). Psychological assessment can serve as a cost-effective solution to such problems. Various risk factors, traits, tendencies, and proclivities can be accurately and rapidly identified for the referring physician by the testing psychologist.

Report Formats in Medical Settings

Eber (1977) indicates six areas in which the intervention of psychological and biological factors should be considered. Testing psychologists may wish to review them and incorporate them into patient formulations and testing reports (p. 177):

1. A description of the patient's lifestyle.
2. Motivational patterns, including areas of energy investment and areas of facilitation.
3. Psychiatric status.
4. Health risk assessment with respect to stress-related disorders, coronary artery disorders, proneness to accidents, presence of self-destructive or self-harming tendencies, and so on.
5. Descriptions of vocational interests.
6. Suggestions regarding ways in which patient cooperation can be enhanced.

For their part, psychologists must write assessment reports that are:

1. Brief (one page preferred, two pages maximum).
2. To the point.
3. Specific.
4. Bulleted.
5. Symptom/diagnosis/treatment-focused.

Long narrative reports are of little pragmatic value to most non-psychiatric physicians. Soliciting feedback from physician-users of such reports will aid in tailoring an appropriate style. These considerations fit most biological disorders or medical complaints that a testing psychologist may evaluate. Automated social histories, as discussed in Chapter 4, can provide rich, helpful data, are self-administered, and are remarkably inexpensive.

Primary Care Psychologist Concept

Wiggins (1994) and Hersch and Staunton (1995) note that clinical psychologists may actually serve as "primary care psychologists." This perspective highlights the fact that psychologists can readily provide diagnostic and therapeutic services for a wide range of disorders. Furthermore, many of the disorders that may initially present to primary care physicians may be better assessed by a psychologist than by a screening conducted by a physician. Exacerbation of a physical illness by co-morbid psychological problems or behavioral issues, or by purely psychological somatoform disorders (Hersch & Staunton, 1995) may also be more accurately diagnosed by using a psychological battery.

Practicing with Physicians:
A Collaborative Model

Testing psychologists working in conjunction with primary care physicians, internists, family practitioners, or other medical specialists need to be sensitive to referral questions and subsequent treatment recommendations. For example, issues of medication or rehabilitation compliance are key in such settings (Hersch & Staunton, 1995).

It is quite helpful for psychologists who provide assessment services to various nonpsychiatric medical specialists and generalists to adopt the perspective of collaborator and healthcare team member. Operationally, this could require providing testing services within a physician's office, a clinic, or a general medical/surgical hospital. For some psychologists, this may seem awkward at first, but there is no reason for discomfort. No longer are such venues the sole locale of health psychologists or medical psychotherapists. Testing psychologists need to realize the pragmatic demands and current circumstances of today's healthcare system. One of these realizations focuses on HMO-based primary care physicians' wish to maximize their levels of productivity. PCPs cannot spend inordinate amounts of time with patients who are inappropriately utilizing their clinical time. Testing psychologists can offer services that more rapidly identify such cases and aid in triage and referral to more therapeutic modes of care. From both a marketing perspective and a clinical perspective, earlier identification and referral provide maximum clinical benefit for the patient in tandem with expeditious referral *out of* inappropriate care (e.g., psychological/psychiatric as opposed to general practice).

The "Generalist" Testing Psychologist

From a marketing perspective, early identification and referral also provide the notable benefits of enhancing "compliance with physician recommendations, [addressing] the stress and behavioral contributions to the illness, and possibly [preventing] some bona fide mental illness from emerging" (Hersch & Staunton, 1995, p. 19). It is important for testing psychologists to adopt the role of generalists. A good collaborative relationship between a testing psychologist and a physician may require the testing psychologist to think like an interventionist in order to perform these services:

1. Aiding in the communication of test results to the patient or family.
2. Constructing behavior modification plans for enhancing treatment and/or medication compliance.
3. Aiding with psychosomatic illnesses.
4. Helping patients and families cope with a debilitating disease or chronic disorder.
5. Consulting for medically mandated lifestyle changes (e.g., diet, smoking cessation).
6. Assisting a patient and family who must cope with news of a fatal disease diagnosis.

Operationally, these services could be conducted via psychoeducational "classes," support groups, individual and family therapy, and/or joint meetings with the patient/family, with a physician or nurse present.

COLLABORATIONS AND PRACTICE ENHANCEMENT

Adaptive, collaborative models shared by psychologists and physicians are key areas of growth and expansion as managed care evolves to more capitated, all-inclusive, and carve-in models (i.e., benefit designs that *include* behavioral healthcare services). These additional areas of psychological evaluation and consultation should be considered for practice expansion:

1. Smoking cessation.
2. Drug abuse.
3. Drug dependence.
4. Alcoholism.
5. Obesity.
6. Anorexia.
7. Bulimia.
8. Headache.
9. Sleep disorders.
10. Type A health-risk behaviors.
11. Kidney dialysis.
12. Chemotherapy and a cancer diagnosis.
13. Terminal disease counseling: patient.
14. Terminal disease counseling: family/significant other(s).
15. HIV-positive.
16. Hospice consultation.
17. Diabetes.
18. Arthritis.
19. Postaccident/trauma recovery.
20. Seizure disorder.
21. Gastrointestinal disorders (e.g., ulcers, irritable bowel).
22. Hypertension.
23. Poststroke rehabilitation.
24. Exercise and diet compliance.
25. Geropsychiatric issues (e.g., Alzheimer's, Pick's, sexual dysfunction, incontinence).
26. Stress/lifestyle alteration and coping.
27. Psychoneuroimmunological issues.
28. Cardiac problems.
29. Prevention of disease/recurrence.
30. Differential diagnosis between psychological and biological disorders.
31. Chronic pain.
32. Burn recovery (skin grafts, motor facility retraining).

33. Menopausal transition.
34. Spinal cord injuries and adaptation/coping.
35. Asthma and respiratory disorders.
36. Obstetrics (prelabor and delivery relaxation, postpartum depression).
37. Degenerative disorders.
38. Surgery preparation/recovery.
39. Lupus/collagen vascular diseases.

ALLIED HEALTH PROFESSIONALS

Other allied healthcare professionals can be enlisted by psychologists to provide consultation to their patients (Hersch & Staunton, 1995). Possibilities include evaluation, motivation, and management assistance for physical therapy patients with concomitant or co-morbid psychological concerns; or, dental patients with phobias, anxiety, or somatic concerns. Audiologists, speech pathologists, and occupational therapists (p. 21) might be brought in, as appropriate.

INTEGRATION

Psychology as a profession is moving toward a more fully integrated subspecialty by interfacing with medical patients. A recent example is evident in Harvard Medical School's Polun Institute, which focuses on training, continuing education, and research in the areas of short-term medical crisis counseling and coping with long term-illness—the "loss of control, loss of self-image, dependency, stigma, anger, abandonment, isolation, and death" (McCarthy, 1995, p. 10).

FUNDING AND MANAGED CARE

In consideration of funding for such collaborative models, Kelleher (1995) is optimistic that supportive financial incentives will be developed by managed care companies, especially within capitated payment models. He believes that "managed care arrangements are likely to produce more integrated provider networks . . . [and] increasingly rely on practice guidelines or parameters for the care of patients with mental disorders. Gatekeeping primary care physicians are likely to discourage 'doctor shopping' and duplication of testing as well as reducing emergency department use for non-emergent care" (p. 4).

INTEROFFICE ARRANGEMENTS

Within this type of collaborative model, the physicians who are using such consultation may wish to have the psychologist provide on-site services at their medical offices (Hersch & Staunton, 1995). Doing so is quite beneficial, in many ways. First, it is convenient for the patient, which is a key utilization factor. Second, referrals to the psychologist will increase as he or she becomes considered part of the clinical team. As others within the medical practice come to know, understand, and respect the psychologist for his or her skills and offerings, and as a person, it can reasonably be presumed that a concomitant increase in referrals for evaluation and consultation, where indicated, should follow.

Third, on-site arrangements may be more cost-effective because they decrease the overhead expenses of a typical practice (support staff, office rent and utilities, furnishings, and so forth). However, such economies may not be manifest in all circumstances because practice designs vary. Psychologists who have support staff and work full-time within their own office would likely not realize cost savings from an on-site clinic or medical office arrangement. Instead, it might only serve as a new referral source. There is also a risk of safe harbor violations. It is illegal to receive any type of "compensation" (which would include free office space or support staff) in conjunction with any federally reimbursed (e.g., Medicare) patient service. (See Chapter 7 for a more detailed examination of such risks.) If a practice does not serve Medicare patients, these federal concerns are mitigated. Nevertheless, all contracts, reimbursement models, audit trails, and other verifiable documents must state very clearly that any expense-sharing arrangement complies with all applicable regulatory requirements for disclosure. (An example would be a sublease agreement to pay X dollars for Y square feet of office space being used—where such costs are within the fair market value of the geographic location—along with a reasonable fee paid for support services such as telephone, typing, billing, and so on.)

Practice Expansion

Krug (1977) long ago noted how self-administered psychological tests are valuable and cost-effective sources of diagnostic information for physicians. Time demands decrease for physicians and their assistants, and, simultaneously, they receive rich, helpful information on a patient's psychological and medical status. This is increasingly important because managed care demands more care for less reimbursement, and the practice of medicine is currently marked by risk of malpractice claims, suits, and litigation.

Cattell (1977) notes that "since the days of Hippocrates, discerning physicians have recognized the close relationship between the personality makeup of their patients and the diseases those patients contract. A major challenge of modern clinical medicine lies in the fact that for a specific pathological condition, the presenting symptoms, treatment, results of treatment, and prognosis are as varied as the patients' personality dynamics and socioeconomic milieu" (p. 11). Such a perspective is key to psychology's evaluative role and function within medicine, not only within primary care venues but also with specialties.

Studies of primary care physicians' practice patterns and compositions have demonstrated for over twenty years (Werkman, Mallory, & Harris, 1976) that approximately a third of a typical practice is devoted to the diagnosis and care of patients with psychological or psychosomatic problems. An informal survey of medical specialists uncovered similar conclusions. Table 2.2 (Cattell, 1977; reprinted with permission) is provided as a checklist for psychologists interested in linking their skills to various medical specialists. The table notes the types of disorders that psychologists can clinically impact.

TABLE 2.2
Medical Specialties/Specialists and Disorders with Psychological
Assessment Intervention Potentials

Medical Specialties/Specialists	Disorder Considered Causal/Linked to/Exacerbated by/Correlated to Psychological Conditions
Allergists	Urticaria Asthma
Cardiologists	Hypertension Myocardial Ischemic Disease (related to chronic tension or anxiety states)
Dermatologists	Urticaria Eczema Neurodermatitis Factitious Dermatitis
Endocrinologists	Functional Hypoglycemia Functional Amenorrhea Idiopathic Edema Hypothyroidism Hyperthyroidism Cushing's Disease Addison's Disease
Gastroenterologists	Peptic Ulcers Spastic Colon Ulcerative Colitis Regional Enteritis Crohn's Disease Regional Enteritis Proctitis
Hematologists	Leukemia
Neurologists	Headaches Migraines Local Paralysis Anesthesia Neurasthenia Vertigo Narcolepsy
Oncologists	Reactive Depression Reactive Anxiety

(continued)

TABLE 2.2   (Continued)

Medical Specialties/Specialists	Disorder Considered Causal/Linked to/Exacerbated by/Correlated to Psychological Conditions
Pediatricians	Headaches Stomach Aches Chest Pains Tics Recurrent Vomiting Anxiety Phobias Ubiquitous Acne Substance Abuse
Pulmonary Medicine	Asthma Hyperventilation Syndromes (secondary to anxiety) Emphysema Symptom Exacerbation (secondary to anxiety)
Rheumatologists	Rheumatoid Arthritis Fibrositis Muscular Spasm Conditions
Surgeons	Peptic Ulcers Hiatal Hernias Breast Pain (usually of cystic mastitis origin) Pancreatitis (secondary to alcoholism)
Dentists	Bruxism (secondary to stress) Periodontal Disease (secondary to stress) Lichen Planus
Gynecologists	Pelvic Pain Menstrual Irregularities Menstrual Pain
Obstetricians	Conduct of Labor Ambivalence toward Newborn Postpartum Depression/Psychosis
Ear, Nose, and Throat Specialists	Globus Hystericus Ménière's Disease
Peripheral Vascular Surgeons	Dizziness Vertigo

TABLE 2.2 (Continued)

Medical Specialties/Specialists	Disorder Considered Causal/Linked to/Exacerbated by/Correlated to Psychological Conditions
Plastic Surgeons	Body Dysmorphic Disorders Self-Image Problems Self-Esteem Issues
Thoracic Surgeons	Dysphagia Globus Hystericus
Urologists	Urinary Frequency Enuresis Impotence Genitalia Surgery Genitalia Injury
Anesthesiologists	Preoperative Drug Withdrawal Postoperative Drug Withdrawal Altered Mental Status and Mood
Orthopedic Surgeons	Neck and Back Pain (with a focus on paraspinal musculature; secondary to anxiety, depression, hostility, and dependency)

Adapted from "The Role of Trait Assessment in Clinical Medicine" by Hereward S. Cattell. In Samuel E. Krug (Ed.), Psychological Assessment in Medicine, 1977, pp. 16–19. Champaign, IL: Institute for Personality and Ability Testing, Inc.

In marketing psychological services to medical specialists, psychologists must communicate the reciprocity between medical conditions and psychological status, along with the causal importance of psychological factors in medical/surgical outcome and prognosis. The use of psychological evaluation in the decision-making process is marked—for example, when deciding whether a surgical procedure should be conducted, or determining what level of compliance can be expected with a medication or treatment regimen. (Additional considerations of medical specialties are noted in Chapter 8.)

Practice Expansion with Psychiatrists

Managed care companies are becoming more prescriptive with psychiatrists' medication decisions. Some require a history of medication failure or significant medical contraindications prior to prescribing some psychotropics. The use of psychological personality trait tests as a method to estimate maximum therapeutic response to antidepressant medication in treating clinical depression may thus be a new market for testing psychologists. Neal (1977) noted that a formula using scores on three scales (H, Q_2, Q_3) of the 16 Personality Factors test (16 PF) could predict which depressed patients would respond better to imipramine or to amitriptyline at an overall conformance level of 86.5%. In today's managed care environment, such considerations could be used to treat a depressed patient (without suicidal ideation) solely on an outpatient basis. This approach could maximize the likelihood for therapeutic response within a much shorter time span, while minimizing the side effects (there is greater risk of side effects if more medications need to be tried). The result is improved quality in patient care, with less cost. Such positive impact, which is especially important today, further supports the inclusion of reimbursement for psychological testing as providing real cost savings and as a method of quality enhancement of patient care.

Conclusion

Psychology, especially the activities of testing and assessment, plays a key role in services with medical patients. Currently, various instruments and practice models allow testing psychologists to expand their practice into an area of great need. In doing so, patients and physicians will benefit from psychology's offerings.

CHAPTER 3

Working with Medical Populations

THROUGHOUT THIS BOOK, there is often an unavoidable overlap of concepts. Just as it is difficult to discuss outcomes without also discussing quality management, it is difficult to discretely examine various special population issues without some overlap with primary care, medical cost offset, and other topics that serve as focal chapters herein.

This chapter covers some broad and diverse populations that may be atypical to the testing psychologist or may hold special concerns within a managed care payor environment. The chapter reviews:

1. Depression.
2. Malingering.
3. Chronic pain.
4. Irritable bowel.
5. Geriatric population.
6. Oral surgery.
7. Differential psychodiagnostics (with medical etiologies mimicking psychological disorders).

Author's Note: As with any test, the potential user has the responsibility to be appropriately trained in the use of that test and has a duty to be fully informed as to the limitations, applications, strengths, weaknesses, normative population, reliability, and validity of any tests used. This author neither endorses nor critiques any commercially available test in this book, but, instead, simply lists relevant information sufficient to provide the reader with guidance to learn more about any testing tool available.

This chapter cannot be exhaustive nor is it meant to be. It provides an overview of diagnostic categories that are felt to have specific relation to special testing issues and considerations within a managed care environment.

Depression

Most testing psychologists are well aware of depression and its clinical manifestation. However, some may not be equally conversant with: the variety of specific screening tools available, co-morbidity with other medical disorders, or causal medication side effects. Depression is highly prevalent, yet it is often undiagnosed by nonbehavioral healthcare specialists.

The U.S. Department of Health and Human Services has sponsored a Depression Guideline Panel. The following focus on depression is based on one of the Panel's public domain documents. Readers interested in this booklet, or other titles in the guideline series, should contact the Agency for Health Care Policy and Research (AHCPR), Executive Office Center, Suite 401, 2101 E. Jefferson Street, Rockville, MD 20852, and request Publication No. 93.0550, *Depression in Primary Care: Volume 1. Detection and Diagnosis.* This guideline is the result of a tremendous clinical/research effort and exhaustive literature review by some of the top clinicians in the country. (Excerpts herein are reproduced with permission.)

WHY TEST FOR DEPRESSION?

It is unlikely that an individual would be referred for a psychological battery to rule in or rule out a depressive disorder. The referral would not be clinically or fiscally efficient and would probably not be approved by a utilization reviewer or managed care company. Depression may become manifest through use of the MMPI-2, Millon Clinical Multiaxial Inventory-Third Edition (MCMI-III), or SCL-90-R, for instance, but such instruments may be too costly or take too much time if the only diagnostic search is for depression. Many mental health professionals are quite comfortable with diagnoses of depression without utilizing such instruments. When a case is more complex or when a patient is not already receiving care from a mental health professional, testing instruments, batteries, or screening tools become necessary. For example, a modified Halstead-Reitan neuropsychological battery would be very useful in differentiating clinical depression from dementia. (This example is amplified later in the chapter.)

TESTING LIMITATIONS

Limitations to using standardized objective tests such as the MMPI do exist in certain differential psychodiagnostic circumstances. Donnelly, Murphy, and Goodwin (1976) found that the MMPI profiles of patient-subjects with major depression displayed elevations across almost all the clinical scales when compared to bipolar, depressive-phase cohorts. This finding is controversial, however, because others (Lumry, 1978; Silver, Isaacs, & Mansky, 1981) have failed to replicate it. The MMPI is also not seen as being appropriate as a "sole means to determine if a patient with a concurrent symptomatic nonpsychiatric medical illness 'really' has depression, because symptoms from the medical illness itself affect test results" (AHCPR, 1993, p. 82). Testing psychologists familiar with MMPI test results of medical patients will likely recognize this occurrence, because these patients' data typically display a two-point elevation on depression and hypochondriasis. The elevation results from the MMPI's sensitivity to "somatic symptoms that emanate from nonpsychiatric medical illness contributing to the depressive/hypochondriacal symptom scales" (AHCPR, 1993, p. 82). Thus, caution and marked clinical judgment must be used by psychologists when selecting tests and interpreting data received from such populations, to achieve maximal differential psychodiagnostic accuracy.

APPROPRIATE INSTRUMENT SELECTION

Most clinically sophisticated managed care organizations or utilization reviewers will be aware of these issues and limitations. Psychologists must be equally aware of them and must recognize the appropriate opportunity to select instruments for specific purposes. Thus, when the referral objective is to differentiate between a depressive disorder and a non-anxiety-related psychiatric condition, or to provide a differential psychodiagnosis, an appropriately constructed battery or selected objective testing instrument may be clinically merited. But use of such protocols, batteries, or tests for general screening is not likely to be approved by managed care organizations, nor is it good practice.

PATIENT SELF-REPORT SURVEYS

The AHCPR (1993) notes that various self-administered report surveys provide a low-cost, valuable, easily administered, case-finding way to aid clinicians not trained in behavioral health to better identify depressed patients (for example, in primary care settings). Such instruments (for samples, see Beckham & Leber, 1985; Marsella, Hirschfeld, & Katz, 1987) provide ease of completion by the patient as well as ease of scoring/use by the practitioner. Often, such surveys are given to medical patients to complete in waiting rooms, as a rule-out precursor to medical diagnosis and treatment planning. The data they yield are not psychodiagnostic by any means, but they may provide an indication for further consultation or evaluation by a psychologist.

Coulehan, Schulberg, and Block (1989, as cited in AHCPR, 1993) noted that the four most common self-report questionnaires used in ambulatory medical settings are:

1. General Health Questionnaire (GHQ).
2. Center for Epidemiological Studies—Depression Scale (CES-D).
3. Beck Depression Inventory (BDI).
4. Zung Self-Rating Depression Scale (ZSRDS).

All of these screens provide direction as to whether further psychodiagnostic evaluation should be conducted. Users should be wary that these screens hold false-positive rates as high as 25% to 40%, but few false negatives.

SELF-REPORT SURVEY SELECTION

The AHCPR (1993) recommends following three guidelines when considering self-report survey selection based on the findings in the literature (pp. 76–77):

1. Because the positive predictive value of self-report questionnaires relates to the prevalence of the disorder in the clinical population, depression scales are most appropriately and efficiently administered to those at higher risk for this disorder. This group includes patients with:

   a. Disabling chronic diseases.
   b. Unexplained or ill-defined symptoms.
   c. Sleep complaints.
   d. History of prior psychiatric illness.
   e. Headaches.
   f. Abdominal pain.
   g. Other pain complaints.
   h. A sad mood or reduced interest or pleasure (anhedonia).

2. Cutoff thresholds for each questionnaire must be established at levels specific to primary care populations. Because positive predictive value is linked to the disorder's prevalence, the threshold most appropriate to particular medical patient groups differs from that to be used with psychiatric or community cohorts. Several investigators have recommended that significantly higher cutoff scores be used with self-report instruments in medical practices, to reduce the proportion of false positives produced by cutoff scores established in community studies (Schulberg et al., 1985; Turner & Romano, 1984). If the practitioner is already highly attuned to and inquires regularly about depressive symptoms, the self-reports may add little to his or her practice.

3. These questionnaires identify patients as "depressed" when they have only some symptoms, but not the disorder. The practitioner should therefore not rely exclusively on them to make a diagnosis of depressive disorder.

Dobson (1985) found that self-report symptom ratings yield poor divergent validity in discriminating between depression and anxiety. Thus, self-report measures should not be used in such a fashion.

CLINICIAN RATING SCALES

In addition to self-report measures, the literature is filled with various clinician rating scales, such as:

1. Beck-Rafaelsen Depression Scale (BRDS; Beck, Kastrup, & Rafaelson, 1986).
2. Hamilton Rating Scale for Depression (HRS-D; Hamilton, 1968).
3. Inventory for Depressive Symptomatology—Clinical Rated (IDS-C; Rush et al., 1986).
4. Montgomery-Asberg Depression Rating Scale (MADRS; Montgomery & Asberg, 1979).
5. Present State Examination (PSE; Wing, Birley, Cooper, Graham, & Isaacs, 1967).
6. Schedule for Affective Disorders and Schizophrenia (SADS; Endicott & Spitzer, 1978).

MODEL PROTOCOL

Use of these tools in tandem with self-report measures may prove to be cost-efficient and diagnostically effective. With this in mind, the following protocol may prove helpful (AHCPR, 1993, p. 77):

1. Self-report questionnaires can be used to identify those *unlikely* to have major depressive disorder as well. No further questioning or evaluation need be performed with these patients.

2. The condition of those who have significant depressive symptoms based on a self-report should be further evaluated by clinical interview to determine whether the symptoms are of sufficient intensity, number, and duration to meet the criteria for major depressive disorder (or another mood disorder) according to DSM-IV.

3. Some patients who meet the criteria for major depressive disorder, but have a very mild condition (not chronic, psychotic, significantly disabling, or suicidal), may either begin treatment or wait for a reevaluation of their condition in one to two weeks before starting specific treatment, since some 15% to 25% (or higher) of these patients respond to supportive care from the practitioner. Should the patient respond fully to supportive care, the practitioner is advised to see the patient again, as some patients' symptoms may return.

4. Those whose major depressive symptomatology is persistent, disabling, or moderate to severe should be treated. Those with moderate to severe symptoms, in a prolonged depressive episode, or with recurrent episodes with poor interepisodic recovery are *less* likely to respond to clinical management and reassurance alone, and specialty treatment should not be delayed.

DIFFERENTIAL DIAGNOSIS: MODERN PROTOCOL

In terms of the differential diagnosis of depressive disorders, this protocol should prove useful (AHCPR, 1993, p. 78):

1. Conduct a clinical interview to assess the patient of the nine specific signs/symptoms of major depressive disorder according to DSM-IV. This step is essential, since the evidence for the efficacy of various treatments of major depressive disorder is very strong, but is relatively unstudied for nonmajor forms of depression or for dysthymic disorder without a history of major depressive disorder.

2. Interview the patient to investigate the possibility of concurrent substance or alcohol abuse and current use of medications that may cause depressive symptomatology.

3. Conduct a medical review of systems to detect the existence of medical disorders that may biologically cause or be commonly associated with depressive symptoms.

4. Interview the patient further to detect the presence of another concurrent nonmood psychiatric condition that may be associated with and be responsible for the depressive symptoms.

5. Exclude alternative causes (1 through 4) for depressive symptoms or syndromes to diagnose a primary mood disorder.

These procedures add to patient care while concomitantly serving as a cost-effective means of quality accurate assessment, which acts to reduce overall care costs. These benefits are important and should be communicated to payors, HMOs, and managed care organizations.

CONTRIBUTORY PATIENT RISK FACTORS FOR DEPRESSION

The following risk factors are not related to test data, but psychologists should generally take them into consideration during the diagnostic process (AHCPR, 1993, pp. 73–74):

1. Prior episodes of depression.
2. Family history of depressive disorders.
3. Prior suicide attempt.
4. Female gender.
5. Age of onset under 40.
6. Postpartum period.
7. Medical co-morbidity.
8. Lack of social support.
9. Stressful life events.
10. Current alcohol or substance abuse.

SUICIDAL RISK FACTORS

Suicidal attempts are more likely among mood-disordered patients, for whom these additional risk factors are present:

1. Hopelessness.
2. Physical illnesses.

3. Family history of substance abuse.
4. Caucasian race.
5. Depression.
6. Substance abuse.
7. Male gender.
8. Advanced age.
9. Presence of psychotic symptoms.
10. Living alone.

Testing psychologists using these criteria may find them persuasive when requesting managed care organizations to approve further psychological testing, additional outpatient sessions, or perhaps admission for necessary inpatient care.

CONFOUNDING MEDICATION EFFECTS

Depressive symptomatology may be associated with a variety of side effects of prescription medications. Psychologists do not prescribe medications, but it is important for them to have an understanding of any medications that may be associated with depressive manifestations. The following list is offered as a handy reference for testing psychologists who must conduct a clinical interview or a chart review:

1. Cardiovascular drugs:
   Alpha-methyldopa.
   Clonidine.
   Digitalis.
   Guanethidine.
   Propranolol.
   Reserpine.
   Thiazide diuretics.
2. Hormones:
   ACTH (corticotropin) and gluococorticoids.
   Anabolic steroids.
   Oral contraceptives.

3. Psychotropics:
   Benzodiazepines.
   Neuroleptics.
4. Anti-Inflammatory/Anti-Infective Agents:
   Ethambutol.
   Metoclopramide.
   Nonsteroidal anti-inflammatory agents.
   Sulfonamides.
5. Others:
   Amphetamines (withdrawal).
   Baclofen.
   Cimetidine.
   Cocaine (withdrawal).
   Cycloserine.
   Disulfram.
   L-dopa.
   Ranitidine.

These medications have been reported to induce depression in some cases. Not every patient taking one of these medications will necessarily be depressed. The cause of depression in a depressed person receiving medical/pharmacological treatment is not necessarily the medication. This list is provided as a heuristic guide to indicate that certain medications should be evaluated as *possible* causes of depression in particular patients.

CONFOUNDING MEDICAL CONDITIONS

In a later section, this chapter examines issues and methodologies of the differential diagnostic process when a variety of psychiatric-mimicking medical disorders are present. As for depression per se, several medical diagnostic categories must be distinguished in order to achieve psychodiagnostic accuracy. Knowledge of the following medical conditions will aid in more fully evaluating diagnostic issues (AHCPR, 1993, pp. 56–65):

Stroke

Guideline: Depression following stroke is not fully explained as a psychological response to the associated impairment. There appear to be subgroups of depressed poststroke patients whose depression is causally related to the injury, possibly including: its strategic location in the brain (left dorsal-lateral frontal cortex or left basal ganglia); a family history of depression; premorbid subcortical atrophy; and premorbid or ongoing social factors. When a patient who has recently suffered a stroke meets the criteria for a major depressive episode, organic (secondary) mood disorder is then diagnosed.

Dementia

Guideline: When patients present with signs of both depression and dementia and the symptoms suggestive of dementia are significantly more prominent, the diagnosis is "dementia with depressive symptoms." If symptoms suggesting a major depressive episode are at least as prominent as those consistent with dementia, the diagnosis is "major depressive disorder." When selecting treatment, it is prudent to assume, until proven otherwise, that the symptoms suggesting dementia may be manifestations of the depressive disorder. When the depressive episode ends, so should the symptoms suggestive of dementia. If they do not, the diagnosis of early dementia should be entertained.

Depressive symptoms are associated with both cortical and subcortical dementing disorders.

Depression is often seen in patients with and/or antecedent to primary dementia.

Diabetes

Guideline: The symptomatic expression of depression in patients with diabetes is analogous to that in patients without diabetes. Given the impact of depression on the management of diabetes and the fact that most diabetic patients do not develop major depression, the practitioner is advised to screen, fully assess, and treat major depression when present in these patients.

Coronary Artery Disease

Guideline: The relationship between depression and increased morbidity and mortality is well documented in both postmyocardial infarction patients and in coronary artery disease patients without myocardial infarction. Given the higher morbidity and the fact that most of these patients do not develop a major depression, it is advisable to screen, fully assess, and treat major depression if it is present within these patients.

Cancer

Guideline: It is essential to separate the symptoms of cancer or its treatment from those of a depressive disorder. A history and clinical interview are needed for a definitive diagnosis. The symptoms of persistent dysphoria, feelings of helplessness and worthlessness, loss of self-esteem, and wishes to die are the most reliable indicators of clinical depression in patients with cancer. Because major depression occurs in approximately 25% of patients with cancer, it should be independently diagnosed and treated.

Risk factors with cancer patients should be given primary attention. The following risk factors predispose cancer patients to develop depressive disorders:

1. Social isolation.
2. Recent losses.
3. A tendency to pessimism.
4. Socioeconomic pressures.
5. A history of mood disorder.
6. Alcohol or substance abuse.
7. Previous suicide attempt(s).
8. Poorly controlled pain.

Suicide risk among cancer patients requires assessment of any depressed patient with cancer. Suicidal risk factors include:

1. A prior psychiatric diagnosis (especially depression).
2. Increasing age.

3. Family history of suicide.
4. Poor social support.
5. Delirium.
6. Advanced stage of disease.
7. Disfiguring disease or surgery.
8. Substance abuse.
9. Poorly controlled pain.

Chronic Fatigue Syndrome

Guideline: Nearly all depressed patients complain of fatigue and low energy. This symptom is associated with a 46% to 75% lifetime rate of major depressive disorder (AHCPR, 1993 pp. 64–65). Complaints of chronic fatigue must be differentiated from the formal chronic fatigue syndrome (CFS). The key feature of CFS is persistent and excessive fatigability. Along with this would be some combination of aching muscles and joints, headache, sore throat, painful lymph nodes, muscle weakness, sleep disturbance, mental fatigue, labile moods, poor concentration, and dysthymia (AHCPR, 1993, p. 64).

Fibromyalgia

This common, nonspecific illness is characterized by muscle pain, soreness, or tenderness. It may involve any fibromuscular tissue, but it typically involves the lumbar region, neck, shoulders, thorax, and thighs.

Guideline: As with other medical conditions, patients with fibromyalgia may or may not have clinical depression. If present, it should be diagnosed and treated as a separate entity.

A Graphic Decision Model

Figure 3.1 is offered as a graphic aid in determining major depression versus other mimicking biological disorders.

Malingering

Managed care companies declare as their mission the adequate management of behavioral health care utilization at the most appropriate

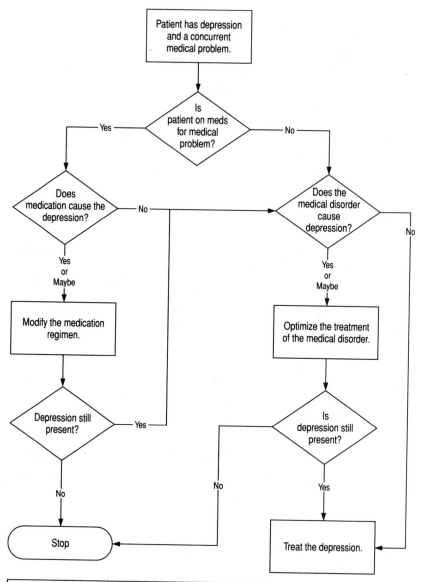

FIGURE 3.1
Graphical Decision Model

level. Previous portions of this book have discussed various disorders and settings that benefit from the accurate assessment of a behavioral health problem. This subsection takes a slightly different but perhaps more powerful perspective on the use of various psychological and neuropsychological tests (and now, technologies) in the unmasking of patients who are malingering.

Managed care organizations (and any other payors, for that matter—e.g., workers' compensation, court or legal judgments/settlements) are extremely interested in psychologically based methodologies that can determine whether an individual is indeed feigning a disorder (for secondary gains or because of a psychopathological etiology, such as Factitious Disorder) and thus inappropriately utilizing clinical services and increasing wasteful expenditures or unnecessary care. Undiagnosed malingering within medical healthcare can result in enormous increases in costs for payors. For managed care organizations, the expertise of psychologists is the key to unmasking such cases.

MALINGERING "STRATEGIES"

Beetar and Williams (1995, pp. 60–61) note that various "strategies" may be employed by individuals wishing to provide intentionally erroneous data. These strategies are presented in Table 3.1.

Beetar and Williams (1995) also examined symptom validity measures such as:

1. Memorization of 15 Items Test (Rey, 1964).
2. Dot Counting: Grouped and Ungrouped (Rey, 1941).
3. Letters and Numbers Task (Binder & Pankratz, 1987; Hiscock & Hiscock, 1989).

Their examination was conducted in tandem with a battery composed of the Memory Assessment Scales (Williams, 1991) with all of the subtests:

1. List learning.
2. Prose memory.

TABLE 3.1
"Strategies" to Provide Erroneous Data

Malingering Strategy	Test(s) to Uncover	Study	Malingering Findings	True Positive
Random responding	Speech-sounds perception test	Heaton, Smith, Lehman, & Vogt, 1978	Depressed scores with worse-than-chance results	Performance not worse than chance
Intentional wrong responses	Various forced-choice symptom validity tests	Goebel, 1983 Hiscock & Hiscock, 1989	Worse-than-chance performance	N/A
Delayed responding	Various motor performance tasks (e.g., Block Design, Object Assembly subtests of WAIS-R)	Goebel, 1983 Resnick, 1984	Response latency	Slow responding across a variety of measures, including untimed
Inattentiveness	Memory assessment scales	Williams, 1991	Immediate recall performance scores within same range as consolidation measures; any poorer performance on visual recognition measures than on visual recall measures	More consistency with intratest similarity measuring scales

3. Delayed list recall.
4. Verbal span.
5. Visual span.
6. Visual recognition.
7. Visual reproduction.
8. Names–faces learning.
9. Delayed list recall.

10. Delayed prose memory.
11. Delayed visual recognition.
12. Delayed names–faces recall.

Beetar and Williams were still unable to detect significant malingering among subjects who might have been purposely faking subtests. They argue that psychological and neuropsychological tests such as these may indeed be insufficiently sensitive or sophisticated to detect less overt forms of malingering.

New Technologies and Methodologies

CogniSyst, Inc. (919-489-4434) claims that its instrument, Computerized Assessment of Response Bias™—Revised Edition (CARB), provides testing psychologists with "an independent and reliable method of assessing subjects' tendency to 'under-perform,' . . . (and) . . . to aid in the assessment of malingering, conversion, motivation, and other response bias" (advertisement, February, 1995). CogniSyst, Inc. use CARB as a computer-administered forced-choice visual recognition test that assesses reaction times, hand preference, and performance patterns for both correct and incorrect responses. It takes approximately 20 minutes to administer.

Rosenfeld, Ellwanger, and Sweet (in press) have investigated a new dimension in the area of malingered amnesia. This innovative technological approach involves recording, via an electroencephalogram (EEG), event-related evoked potentials, while presenting subjects with various recall and recognition tasks. The EEG data on P300 amplitudes were statistically significant (92% to 93% correct discrimination rates for numeric data presented, and 77% for name data presented). This finding suggests that when a malingering amnesic subject (or patient) is presented with presumably rememberable or known data but denies any such recognition, the EEG data will be immune to faking and will provide a presumably reliable measure of what is and what is not familiar. This "crossover" of the psychological and the neurological is likely to experience continuing, if not expanded, development as the EEG technologies advance along with psychometric methodologies.

Chronic Pain

Eimer (1988) has identified a protocol in the psychological assessment of chronic pain patients. This battery is designed to provide aid to medical practitioners and to treating psychologists (clinical, medical, rehabilitation, or health specialties). Eimer's model is based on Lazarus's (1981) modality profile of the BASIC I.D., which covers seven areas or "modalities":

1. Behavior.
2. Affect.
3. Sensation.
4. Imagery.
5. Cognitions.
6. Interpersonal.
7. Drugs and biology.

(Readers familiar with Lazarus's work with multimodal therapy will recognize this as a general model for also conceptualizing, assessing, and treating psychopathology.) The BASIC I.D. data are obtained via the self-administered multimodal life history questionnaire (Lazarus, 1981). This questionnaire provides a great deal of information concerning the patient's history and demographics. It is remarkably complete and thus may be a bit time-consuming for the patient. It is one of the few instruments that (in most clinical circumstances) a patient can complete at home and return. In many instances, it can serve as a substitute for the clinical time that would be needed to gather personal data and social history. (Use of the multimodal life history questionnaire may be considered standard in some practices or settings. It is sufficiently generalizable to not be limited to its focus on the multimodal approach.) Eimer (1988) additionally recommends the following instruments:

1. Patient Pain Questionnaire (Turk, Meichenbaum, & Genest, 1983).
2. McGill Pain Questionnaire (Melzack, 1975).
3. Beck Depression Inventory (Beck, 1967).

The Behavior Assessment of Pain (BAP), by Tearnan and Lewandowski (1992), is also available by calling 702-828-2955.

These instruments are self-administered, provide rapid scoring, and are cost-effective (i.e., inexpensive to purchase, time-efficient, and yielding good data). These attributes make them "managed care friendly"—a combination that may aid testing psychologists in gaining approval and payment for these and other testing procedures.

The MMPI is also useful in the testing of pain patients. Differential diagnostic profiles of pain patients (to reveal chronicity) are found with evaluations in scale 1 (hypochondriasis) and scale 3 (hysteria) for more recent pain-onset patients. Chronic (longer than six months) pain patients display an elevation on scale 2 (depression) that exceeds scales 1 and 3 (Hendler, 1984). Eimer (1988) notes that patients whose pain has lasted more than three years will show a decline in scale 2 and continued scale 1 and 3 elevations (similar to acute pain patients).

The Symptom Check List-90-Revised (SCL-90-R; Derogatis, 1977) can also be used in this way. Its shorter length of administration and ease of scoring may make it more appealing. Acute pain patients display positive symptom cases for elevations in anxiety and somatization, and patients with increasing duration of pain demonstrate elevations in dimensions of depression and interpersonal sensitivity (Eimer, 1988).

CHRONIC PAIN CASE REPORT MODEL

The issues listed below should be included in a patient's report as standard components. Some issues may not be familiar to some testing psychologists, even those trained within health or medical settings (Eimer, 1988, p. 27):

1. Medical history.
2. Psychiatric history.
3. Precipitating events.
4. Circumstances surrounding pain onset.
5. Characteristics of the pain.

6. Course of the pain episodes over time.
7. Effects of situation and activities on the pain.
8. Related physical symptomatic complaints.
9. Related psychological symptomatic complaints.
10. Patient's own thoughts/theories as to the pain's cause(s).
11. Meanings that may be assigned to the pain's occurrence.
12. Coping methods.
13. Restricted activities.
14. Effect on interpersonal relationships.
15. Indication of motivation for treatment (e.g., willingness to work hard; expectations; considerations/fantasies of how life will differ if without pain).

A well-integrated report, regardless of which tests are used, will likely need to incorporate most of these issues. The testing psychologist must always take into account the referral question(s), the needs (e.g., psychological treatment planning, rehabilitation planning, and so on) and users (e.g., clinical or medical psychologists, physical therapists, physicians, nurses, etc.) of the report, and any other special circumstances of the patient, testing setting, or therapists.

Irritable Bowel

The disorder of irritable bowel syndrome (IBS) is common in 14% to 22% of the general population of the United States (Sandler, Drossman, Nathan, & McKee, 1984). It may be chronic or episodic; it is characterized by abdominal pain without organic etiology. It is also referred to as irritable or spastic colon or as mucous colitis (Jones, 1989). Testing psychologists' screening services have been useful to patients with this disorder and to the physicians treating them.

Both the SCL-90-R and the Millon Behavioral Health Inventory (MBHI) are noted (Jones, 1989) as being useful tools. The SCL-90-R's utility with pain patients, as discussed earlier, is of similar utility with IBS cases. The MBHI provides a specific gastrointestinal susceptibility scale along with interpretive impressions as to which patients may best respond to behavioral interventions or psychopharmacological interventions (Richter, Obrecht, & Laurence, 1986). Additionally, albeit a longer test, the MMPI has been used specifically with IBS patients (Bergeron & Monto, 1985; Bonfils & De M'Uzon, 1974; Esler & Goulston, 1973).

MODEL HISTORY PROTOCOL

As is true with pain patients and other medical patients, the importance of a detailed and tailored history is marked. Jones (1989, p. 16) makes the following recommendations:

1. Present life circumstances:
   General issues.
   Losses.
   Failures.
   Crises.
   Achievements.
   Goals.
2. Detailed description of the problem:
   Frequency.
   Intensity.
   Duration.
   Level of life disruption.
   Effect on:
   Work environment.
   Family environment.
   Social environment.
   Internal/external stressors as they relate to IBS symptoms (exploring for any exacerbations/alleviations).
3. Rule out depression marked by anxiety as evidenced by:
   Sleep disturbance.
   Mood swings.
   Anorexia.
   Fatigue.

Sex drive.
Psychosomatic symptoms.
4. Lifestyle issues:
Social history.
Sexual history.
Eating habits.
Prescription/nonprescription drug use.
Alcohol use.
Caffeine use.
Tobacco use.
Exercise habits.
Hobbies.
5. Historic data:
Parental illness and medical history.
Sibling illness and medical history.
Offspring illness and medical history.
Spouse illness and medical history.

Latimer (1983) suggests the use of a diary or log of some type to track "real time" data of diet, bowel dysfunction, pain, stressors, sleeping patterns, and so on, in order to collect pattern and trend data and, eventually, draw conclusions about causal relationships. This tactic engages the patient in the evaluative process (or draws resistance if the patient is uncooperative). Such findings tend to then generalize to treatment compliance issues. Issues to be considered in the communication of findings parallel those noted in pain patient cases.

Geriatric Population

Geropsychological and geriatric patient populations are an increasing percentage of our national population. Appropriately trained psychologists are likely to see an increase in the testing of these patients. Issues of psychopathology, organic disorders, cognitive degenerative disorders, substance abuse, and grief and loss, will be paramount. These disorders bring along with them the complexity of polypharmacy and physical degenerative disorders, and social changes associated with the aging process.

Psychological batteries, often supplemented with neuropsychological tools, would be used. Instruments that examine general functioning, adaptability, and intellect/cognition are often helpful with this population. In instances where mood or other psychopathologies are absent, the neuropsychological battery, its components, or screens would be used. Currently, most managed care organizations are not tooled-up for heavy utilization by an aged patient population. But this surely will change, based on the demographics of covered lives. In the meantime, Medicare provider psychologists can conduct neuropsychological as well as psychological testing for Medicare patients. Various Current Procedural Terminology (CPT) codes (which periodically change) are involved as are annual limitations to the amount of time allowed for testing. Thus, it is important for psychologists to first check with a state or regional office in order to accurately provide services within a patient's benefit availability.

Oral Surgery

Psychologists have been collaborating increasingly with oral surgeons and dentists in treatment of phobias, fears, and other dental-related anxieties. One model of testing (Buffone, 1989) includes using the MMPI as an initial screening instrument for gross psychopathology, especially in the areas of anxiety (scale 7), depression (scale 2), paranoia (scale 6), schizophrenia (scale 8), and mania (scale 9). Additionally, the MacAndrew Scale provides insight as to the presence of possible risks in pain medication use such as abuse potential or interference in medication efficacy. Other scales such as an ego strength (ES) scale may provide guidance in a patient's ability to manage stress or change (Buffone, 1989).

"SURGICAL" REPORT MODEL

Most surgeons (as well as other physical medicine specialists) prefer short, concise, specific reports that highlight not only problems but also specific recommendations as to intervention strategies. Some surgeons have "surgical clearance" as the referral question. Testing psychologists' responses to this question typically are one of the following (Buffone, 1989, p. 41):

1. Surgically cleared.
2. Cleared with special considerations.
3. Postponed.
4. Disapproved for surgery.

These items would be expected to be clearly noted and supported within the report. Mitigating factors to surgical procedures could include high presurgery anxiety, poor relationship with the surgeon, or psychosocial conditions that may interfere with postsurgical recovery or adjustment (e.g., high levels of depression) (Buffone, 1989).

Differential Psychodiagnostics

This author has examined the area of medical or biological disorders/etiologies that manifest as psychological in nature in a variety of procedures (Stout, 1988, 1989, 1990, 1994). The risk management issues associated with the misdiagnosis of these disorders are noted in Chapter 7. It seems fitting to close this chapter with an actual methodology and system for users.

Many patients may present to a testing psychologist or other mental healthcare professional with a complaint that may appear purely "psychosocial" on the surface, but may indeed be endocrine in etiology, for example. Testing psychologists must know what to look for and ask about, in order to collect the correct information that will enhance a psychodiagnostic judgment or, more specifically (and thus more cost-effectively), initiate a referral to an appropriate type of specialist.

BIO-PSYCH SCREENING TOOL

Described herein is a set of self-administered forms for a tool called the Bio-Psych Screen™. Its purpose is to gather efficient and expeditious data for testing psychologists. It is described here in its basic form. Testing psychologists' own needs will inevitably produce variations.

The first page (Figure 3.2) collects information on health/lifestyle history and habits. On the next page is a request for information on already diagnosed medical conditions that may exist for the patient. Then follows a broad spectrum of psychiatric symptoms, physical findings, comment on historical physical problems, and observed findings that are symptomatic of more than 20 of the most common medical disorders that present with mimicking psychiatric symptoms. Prior to making a decision on its applicability, a potential user may wish to review the terms to ensure that they are within the reading level of most clientele, or adjust them if necessary.

Symptoms are input to a database that runs a software program available from the author. The program is a database file that receives patient data and searches for associated medical diagnostic categories. It then lists them. If any trend is evident (such as a number of endocrine disorders), the testing psychologist would consider the possibility of a specialist referral to an endocrinologist.

ADDITIONAL USES OF THE BIO-PSYCH SCREEN DATABASE

A testing psychologist may wish to rapidly gain a definition of an unfamiliar medical term used in a history (e.g., bradycardia). Keying the word in a search condition for "definition" would yield the explanation of that word. An expeditious reverse-function use of the database also saves time. If a patient reports a previously confirmed diagnosis of "hypoparathyroidism," the psychologist can input that word to gain a listing of the psychiatric-type symptoms associated with it.

This database is *not* a substitute for consultation or clinical judgment. It is simply a systematized method of rapid data collection and analysis that diminishes the likelihood of missing such information in a clinical interview or social/medical history questionnaire. It also decreases the time that would be required to locate and research definitions or symptom listings via a medical library.

Users of this file must be fluent with database packages; no documentation is provided. (Referral to database software manuals

PSYCHOLOGICAL ASSESSMENT IN MANAGED CARE

Name: _____   Sex: ☐ female ☐ male

ID Number: _____   Race: _____

Date of Birth: _____/_____/_____

- Please list any medications you are currently taking.

  _____

  _____

- Why are you taking the above noted medications?

  _____

  _____

- Have you had any type of injury or accident? If so, please describe.

  _____

  _____

- Have you ever had surgery? If so, please describe.

  _____

  _____

- Please describe your use of the following:

  Alcohol

  _____

  _____

  Non-Prescriptionp medications (e.g., Rolaids, aspirin, Maalox, etc.)

  _____

  _____

  Illicit drugs (e.g., marijuana, cocaine, etc.)

  _____

  _____

  Nicotine

  _____

  _____

  Caffeine

  _____

  _____

  Vitamins

  _____

  _____

  Steroids

  _____

  _____

FIGURE 3.2
Bio-Psych Screen™

Are you currently diagnosed with any of the following disorders (check all that apply):

		When Diagnosed	Medication
☐	Hypoparathyroidism	_____	_____
☐	Hypoadrenalism (Addison's Disease)	_____	_____
☐	Hypothyroidism	_____	_____
☐	Diabetes Mellitus	_____	_____
☐	Early Dementia (Chronic OBS)	_____	_____
☐	Seizure Disorder (Psychomotor or other temporal lobe)	_____	_____
☐	Brain Tumor	_____	_____
☐	Myasthenia Gravis	_____	_____
☐	Delirium (Acute Confusional State or Acute OBS)	_____	_____
☐	Pheochromocytoma (Adrenal Tumor or Carcinoid Tumor)	_____	_____
☐	Subdural Hematoma	_____	_____
☐	Multiple Sclerosis	_____	_____
☐	Pernicious Anemia	_____	_____
☐	Wilson's Disease	_____	_____
☐	Pancreatic Carcinoma	_____	_____
☐	Bacterial Infections	_____	_____
☐	Wernicke's Encephalopathy	_____	_____
☐	Korsakoff's Psychosis	_____	_____
☐	Petiagra (Niacin Deficiency)	_____	_____

Do you have a recent history of, or current problem with:

Psychiatric Symptoms

	Yes	No		Yes	No
Depression	☐	☐	Negativistic	☐	☐
Apathetic	☐	☐	Fear	☐	☐
Anxiety	☐	☐	Panic Attacks	☐	☐
Delusions	☐	☐	Short Attention Span	☐	☐

FIGURE 3.2 (Continued)

	Yes	No		Yes	No
Psychosis	☐	☐	Hallucinations	☐	☐
Confusion	☐	☐	Association Difficulty	☐	☐
Irritability	☐	☐	Concentration Difficulty	☐	☐
Agitation	☐	☐	Social Competence Loss	☐	☐
Acting-Out	☐	☐	Disorientation	☐	☐
Violent Outbursts	☐	☐	Flight of Ideas	☐	☐
Emotional Lability	☐	☐	Unaware of Environment	☐	☐
Automatic Behavior	☐	☐	Personality Disturbance	☐	☐
Suspicious/Paranoid	☐	☐			

Physical Findings

	Yes	No		Yes	No
Hypotension	☐	☐	Hypertension	☐	☐
Tachycardia	☐	☐	Bradycardia	☐	☐
Cardiac Arrythmia	☐	☐	Symtpoms, Heart Disease	☐	☐
Flaccid Quadriplegia	☐	☐	Increased Tendon Reflexes	☐	☐
Visual Gaze Problems	☐	☐	Renal Stones	☐	☐
Loss of Neurological or Muscular Control	☐	☐	Purplish Striate on Abdomen	☐	☐
Cutaneous and Mucosal Pigmentation	☐	☐	Kayser-Fleischer Ring in Cornea	☐	☐
Masses	☐	☐	Fever	☐	☐
Loss of Sex Characteristics in females	☐	☐	Unexplained Physocal Complaints and Findings	☐	☐

Current/History

	Yes	No		Yes	No
Lethargy	☐	☐	Fatigue, Insidious Onset	☐	☐
Amenorrhea	☐	☐	Weakness, Insidious Onset	☐	☐
Fatigue and Weakness, slowly progressive	☐	☐	Decreased Sexual Functioning	☐	☐
Impotence	☐	☐	Decreased Appetite	☐	☐
Decreased Weight	☐	☐	Increased Weight	☐	☐
Abdominal Pain	☐	☐	Recurrent Diarrhea	☐	☐
Constipation	☐	☐	Increased Urination	☐	☐
Urine Odor	☐	☐	Nausea	☐	☐
Vomitting	☐	☐	Salt Craving	☐	☐
Somnolence	☐	☐	Hypersomnia	☐	☐
Head Trauma	☐	☐	Headache	☐	☐
Seizure	☐	☐	Convulsions	☐	☐
Eccentric Food Cravings	☐	☐	Occasional Hypoglycemia	☐	☐
History of Blackouts	☐	☐	Uncoordination	☐	☐

FIGURE 3.2 (Continued)

	Yes	No		Yes	No
Wandering About	☐	☐	Muscle Spasms	☐	☐
Carpopedal Spasms	☐	☐	Fragile Skin	☐	☐
Easy Bruising	☐	☐	Poor Wound Healing	☐	☐
Rash	☐	☐	Dry Skin	☐	☐
Hair Loss	☐	☐	Sweating	☐	☐
Slowing of Intellectual Activity	☐	☐	Heat Intolerance with Excessive Sweating	☐	☐
Cold Intolerance	☐	☐	Stiff Muscles/Aching	☐	☐
Muscle Cramps	☐	☐	Carpal Tunnel Syndrome	☐	☐
Menorrhagia	☐	☐	Osteoporosis	☐	☐
Arthritis	☐	☐	Chest Pain	☐	☐
Inability to Tolerate Significant Exertion	☐	☐	Dyspnea following Exertion	☐	☐
Palpitation	☐	☐	Tetany	☐	☐
Respiratory Paralysis	☐	☐	Diffuse Pain	☐	☐
History of Liver, Renal, or Neurological Disorder	☐	☐	Liver Complaints or Jaundice	☐	☐
Deepening of Voice with Hoarseness	☐	☐	Hearing Deficits	☐	☐

Observed

	Yes	No
Full Facial Expression	☐	☐
Pallor	☐	☐
Moon Fascie	☐	☐
Puffy, Large Tongue	☐	☐
Tremor	☐	☐
Clothes Picking	☐	☐
Periorbital Puffiness	☐	☐
Acne	☐	☐
Lip Smacking	☐	☐
Bad Breath	☐	☐
Unsteady Walking Gait	☐	☐
Pale, Cool Skin, Rough	☐	☐
Incongruent Weight Gain with Central Deposits of Fat, Very Thin Limbs	☐	☐

FIGURE 3.2 (*Continued*)

will resolve most questions.) The database is available free of charge to those who send a 3.5″ formatted DS DD diskette (for DOS systems only); a standard, self-addressed, stamped envelope; and $5.00 to cover copying and handling fees. (Any disks received that do not meet these criteria will be discarded.) This offer is available until January 1, 1998. Materials enclosed with a note requesting this file may be sent to:

> Dr. Chris E. Stout
> c/o Stout Ventures
> 154 Ironwood Court
> Buffalo Grove, IL 60089-6626

Conclusion

Many of the areas discussed in this chapter are not new to testing psychologists; however, they may become a greater proportion of a professional practice and thus should not be neglected. For others, these areas may represent new expansion-of-practice possibilities.

CHAPTER 4

Consulting to Treatment Facilities

THE IMPACT OF CHANGE and the new challenges brought by the advent of managed care in the treatment venues of institutions and facilities parallel practitioners' experiences. It has become equally incumbent for directors and chief executive officers of various care facilities to seek and apply the most cost-effective methods for providing quality care.

Historically, the most rapid means of reducing costs was to decrease services. Today, this is not always practical, even when it may be possible. Quality of care and risk management issues are paramount. Capitated fee arrangements often require various assessments (social histories, psychological testing, outcome study instruments, satisfaction surveys, and so forth) to be conducted. Such circumstances heighten the need to look to efficiencies of time that bring decreases in actual costs.

This chapter focuses on various ways to maintain or improve treatment quality within facilities, while holding costs steady or finding certain economies afforded by assessment and automation. The term "facilities" is used generically to refer to agencies, hospitals, clinics, or any other type of care/treatment venue in which regulatory, contractual, market, and/or patient needs require specific types or a high volume of assessments to be conducted. The examples herein may also hold value for group practices or practices with marked testing volume. Assessment specialists and testing psychologists may also find this chapter useful in developing services or marketing targets where testing arrangements can be provided.

Social Histories

Most inpatient facilities need to collect social history data because of their importance in:

1. The development of treatment plans.
2. The formulation of a context within which to better understand the patient and conceptualize the presenting problem(s) and psychopathology.
3. The exploration of abuse issues or reporting.
4. Identification of other risks.

The procedural flowchart of a traditional social history report is shown in Figure 4.1.

A staff management concern is that the 3.25 to 5.0 hours per patient represent 2.5 to 4.0 hours of staff time taken away from other clinical duties: therapeutic interventions of individual, group, or family treatment; case management activities; treatment planning; clinical liaison; aftercare planning; and other time-intensive activities important to quality patient care.

Typically, a social history would be conducted by a social worker with the patient or an appropriate reporter. Lack of availability of the family (in cases where the patient is a child or adolescent) can make it more difficult to arrange a timely appointment to gather history and report it to the clinical staff for incorporation into the patient's therapeutic activities. When an appointment is made, a social worker needs, on average, 1.5 to 2.5 hours to conduct the interview. After the data are collected, it takes approximately .5 to 1.0 hour to dictate or write the report; another .5 to .75 hour to transcribe it; .25 hour to proof and edit; another .25 hour to type corrections and print out the final draft; and .25 hour to review the final draft. The total time is between 3.25 and 5.0 hours per patient report, and about 2 to 4 days' turnaround time is needed to process and conduct all these activities. If the cost of a staff social worker's time is $22.00 per hour, and a typist's time is $ 9.00, the labor cost (excluding equipment and materials) would range between $61.75 to $97.00 per report. This information is summarized in Table 4.1.

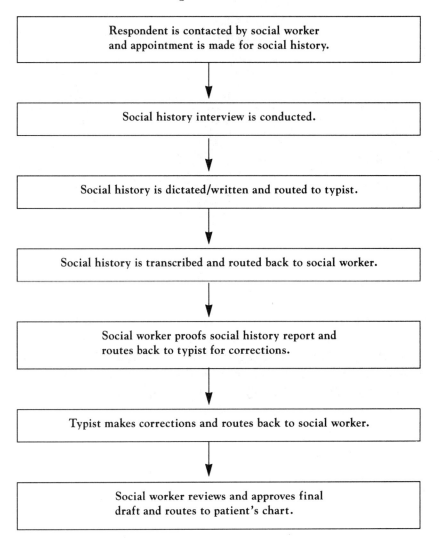

FIGURE 4.1
Social History Procedural Workflow Chart

TABLE 4.1

Labor Costs Associated with Producing a Social History Report

Staff	Hourly Wage	Base Amounts		Possible Range		
		Time (Hours)	Fee	Time (Hours)	Fee	Activity
Social worker	$22.00	1.5	$33.00	2.5	$55.00	Interview
Social worker	22.00	.5	11.00	1.0	22.00	Report dictation
Typist	9.00	.5	4.50	.75	6.75	Transcription
Social worker	22.00	.25	5.50	.25	5.50	Proof/edit
Typist	9.00	.25	2.25	.25	2.25	Type corrections
Social worker	22.00	.25	5.50	.25	5.50	Review final version
Totals		3.25	$61.75	5.00	$97.00	

AUTOMATED SOCIAL HISTORIES

A possible alternative, to ease cost burdens and time constraints, is to use an automated system. The initial systems of this type are the Giannetti On Line Psychosocial History (GOLPH; NCS, 1995) and the Adolescent and Child Automated Social History (ACASH; NCS, 1995). These are computerized programs that have been designed to be interactively administered; that is, the items are displayed on a monitor and the respondent "types in" a response. Very little is actually keyboarded as input/responses.

A CLINICAL MODEL

This author instituted an automated social history system within an inpatient psychiatric facility. Initially (and not unexpectedly), it was met with resistance on the part of the social services staff. The resistance seemed to stem from two concerns: (a) a presumption that respondents would not like to be engaged with a computer program because it seemed too impersonal, and (b) a somewhat guised fear of "being replaced by a machine." Both concerns were understandable. When addressing such changes, administrators must exhibit sensitivity in all stages of planning and implementation, in order to reassure staff members, decrease their fear, and strive to minimize operational resistance.

Involving the social services staff in such a transition is key. They need to understand the economies of time and costs, and to view the introduction of such systems as helpful, rather than a direct threat to their jobs or an implied insult to their professional skills. (In some instances, the social workers may request an automated system and then lobby to persuade the administration to adopt it.) Additionally, a body of scientific literature (Erdman, Klein, & Greist, 1985; Slack & Slack, 1977) indicates that patients are *not* alienated by using a computer. Indeed, research has shown that many patients are actually more honest in their responses to questions posed by computers—a finding that is intuitively supported by clinical realities. If one pictures a 55-year-old male who is being asked about topics that may cause him embarrassment (e.g., sexual activity or deviation; criminal activities or conviction; and so on) by a recently graduated, 23-year-old female social worker, some dishonesty of report may result. Dishonesty could occur with a computer-administered history as well, but it is less likely (Erdman et al., 1985). From a quality perspective, the automated method may actually yield better results.

Additional quality improvements may result from the fact that the computer's performance never varies. It is never distracted by fatigue, illness, a difficult day, a recently manifest crisis, or a negative reaction to the person being interviewed. Most staffs have clinicians who vary in expertise, seniority, style, and focus. Such variations can yield very different social history reports, whereas computer-administered histories are always consistent (but still individualized to each patient). Data are not omitted by decision of the examiner, and differences in skill levels among examiners are not present. Most social services department directors find the benefit of consistency to be very important.

No system is a panacea, and all approaches have drawbacks. Automated programs still require human follow-up to "flagged" items (e.g., abuse reporting or suicidal ideation). Systems may have programming errors ("bugs") or require hardware that may be expensive. In addition, potentially relevant body language, telltale mannerisms, eye contact, and gestures cannot be detected by a computer at this time.

A CLINICAL EXAMPLE

However, the drawbacks of computerized assessment may well be out-weighed by the concomitant time and cost savings. Consider this typical clinical scenario. Upon admission of an adolescent by his or her parents, the psychiatric evaluation and admission paperwork would be completed, and the adolescent would be introduced to the staff and oriented to the unit. While that is occurring, the parents would be invited to complete the automated social history after being fully informed as to their choice between a one-to-one interview with a social worker or an automated interview with the computer. (Policy and procedure would also include a listing of circumstances in which the automated option is not appropriate: illiteracy, vision problems, significant emotional upset, language differences, and so forth.) If the parents choose the automated option, they are escorted to a private, but proctored, office or carrel, and oriented to the sys-tem. Any questions regarding its operation are answered by the ad-mission department staff member (who also would act as proctor, after having been trained), and the testing is initiated. The parents are encouraged to feel free to take breaks, get refreshments, or gener-ally make themselves comfortable.

Upon completion, the program automatically saves the data for scoring. The disk is routed to a person who has been trained and is responsible for "scoring" the disk. The report is produced and re-turned to the social worker for review, signature, and routing to the patient's chart. Any issues that need immediate follow-up are noted in the report, and the social worker and/or primary therapist or psy-chiatrist follows through on them.

This procedure takes approximately .25 hour of the admission de-partment staff member's time, .25 hour of the scoring staff's time, and .25 hour of the social worker's time. If the social worker's time costs $22.00 per hour, admissions staff are paid $10.00 per hour, and scor-ing staff are paid $12.00 per hour, the cost of labor associated with the automated procedure is $11.00. The cost of the program scoring is $7.35 per report, which yields a total cost of $18.35 (see Table 4.2). An additional clinical benefit is that the report can arrive on the unit shortly after the patient's admission, and the social worker has "found"

TABLE 4.2
Costs Associated with Producing a Computerized Social History Report

Staff	Hourly Wage	Activity	Time (Hours)	Amount
Admissions	$10.00	Orient and proctor	.25	$ 2.50
Scoring	12.00	Generate report	.25	3.00
Social worker	22.00	Review report	.25	5.50
		Program fee		7.35
Totals			.75	$18.35

3 to 4.75 more hours per case—time that can be well used to provide other clinical services. Other cost factors to consider here include the computer hardware associated with data collection and scoring. However, this cost can be minimized by using an inexpensive system or programming one computer to administer the history, process the data collected, and report the scoring.

A procedural flowchart for the automated social history report described above is shown in Figure 4.2.

NEW TOOLS

New social history automated methods that will better address logistical and regulatory needs are constantly being developed. The Quick View Basic and Clinical Social History (NCS, 1995) is an example. The Quick View (available only for adults currently) is formatted as a paper-and-pencil survey of historic data. The benefits of this type of format, in lieu of online administration, are that no extra computers are needed or get tied-up in history administration. Some respondents may feel a greater comfort level with the print format, and data collection can be completed privately and comfortably in the patient's room. The answer sheet is computer-scanned, the score is calculated and entered, and a report is rapidly provided for review. New and innovative approaches will most likely be brought to the assessment market by a variety of publishers.

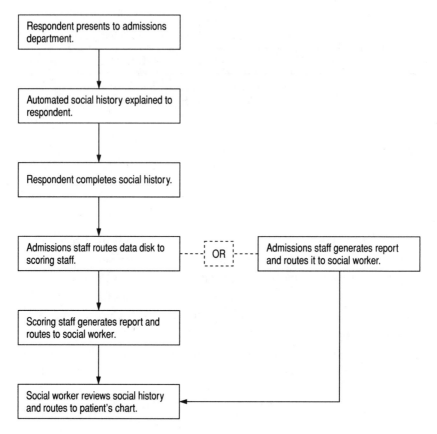

FIGURE 4.2
Automated Social History Procedural Workflow Chart

EVALUATING AUTOMATED TOOLS

As with most instruments or tools, quality of software varies. Before purchasing any software, a potential administrator or clinician user should investigate:

1. What is available.
2. What best fits with the realistic clinical procedures.
3. Needs and operations of the facility.
4. Regulatory requirements that affect patient care.

5. Costs, equipment, and necessary staffing.
6. Development (or alteration) of policies and procedures.
7. Training and evaluation of clinician users and proctors.
8. Planning for acceptance if the staff has a history of resistance to automation.

It is incumbent on psychologists to first learn about a program's psychometric base, the normative sample's database size and composition, and the traditional standard considerations used by psychologists in selecting nonautomated test versions. Other considerations include operating system compatibility (e.g., Apple versus DOS versus Windows versus OS/2 versus UNIX), hardware capability (e.g., hard disk space, network linkages, adequate RAM), training needs, future developments and upgrades (to avoid obsolescence), and system maintenance (both operationally and for data backup/integrity).

The American Psychological Association (APA) has published guidelines for the use, online administration, and scoring of automated tests (Committee on Professional Standards & Committee on Psychological Tests and Assessment, 1986). Automation of psychological practice is more fully discussed in Chapter 9. Individuals interested in automated test administration and scoring should review the APA guidelines in detail.

Additional Testing Opportunities

Facility administrators may wish to incorporate into their systems other types of psychological screening for their clients or patients. Psychologists may find strong markets for their testing services if they appropriately emphasize to behavioral facilities how they may provide numerous benefits by:

1. Improving differential diagnosis.
2. Improving psychodiagnostic accuracy.
3. Uncovering undiagnosed psychopathology.

4. Improving treatment planning.
5. Expediting care via the above benefits.
6. Aiding pre- and posttreatment outcome methodologies.
7. Standardizing screening protocols, to shed light on admission trends, sort patient data according to program development, design staff training and in-service programs, and so on.

Facility administrators would likely be receptive and interested audiences for such improvements. The consulting testing psychologist should take responsibility for learning about the additional needs of the facility and refining a model, plan, or system that will accomplish the identified needs and goals. Automated methods may prove more cost-effective with larger volume demands; however, if demands are small or episodic, there may not be an initial need to use computers in administration or in scoring.

In another variation on this theme, the facility purchases and owns the computers, systems, and/or software for the psychologist's use and then subcontracts with the psychologist to interpret the reports produced, troubleshoot any problems, and perform overseer/manager duties. Such an arrangement is more collaborative and mutually cost-effective for the psychologist (who doesn't have to purchase hardware, software, or usages) and the facility (which doesn't need to hire any additional full-time employees—just a part-time consultant).

Practice Models

Systems vary in their designs. The least expensive unit consists of a test kit (or kits), answer sheets, scoring-by-hand utensils, and a word processor for use in writing the report or findings. However, this least expensive unit is the most time-intensive. A refinement would be to use a mail-in or fax-in service. The patient's completed answer sheets (carrying a number code rather than name and address) would be sent or faxed to a scoring facility. A computer-produced report would be mailed or faxed back within a short (specified) time frame. This scenario decreases the clinician's time but takes a few days of turnaround time, has risks associated with the loss of patient data, and carries confidentiality concerns. Faxing options act to mitigate these risks—if the psychologist has a secure fax machine that can ensure confidentiality.

A third alternative is to utilize electronic transmission of data and return of the report via modem. This is a reasonably secure and quite rapid means of data transfer and receipt, but it requires a computer with a modem and software that supports the file transfer functions. This is not difficult to arrange, but it represents an increase in initial operational costs. If the test was not administered online, then the psychologist must take the time (or hire a data-entry person) to input the patient's responses. Besides the risk of data entry errors, it would be quite tedious (and error-prone) to key in the 567 items of the MMPI-2! The system would allow review of the entered data prior to transmission, in order to manually verify each item. This is a necessary and encouraged procedure, but it takes considerable time.

A final, state-of-the-art system option is available with current technologies: online test administration with on-site data processing, scoring, and report production. If tests yield paper-and-pencil responses, they can be scanned for scoring. This system offers the most rapid turnaround times, ensures patient confidentiality, and diminishes the risk of data or report loss. The primary barrier may be cost; this is the most expensive design. However, multiple tests can be used, multiple tasks or activities can be accomplished with the computer running various programs simultaneously, and rapid information processing capabilities may mitigate the higher cost for many facilities over a remarkably short time.

An Important Caveat

An additional word of caution: psychologists must clearly communicate, to any facility administrators with whom they may work, that computerized psychological tests are meant to be evaluated by *appropriately trained* psychologists. There may be a predisposition on the administrator's part to view computerized assessment as something that requires only a computer, not a psychologist. This view does not necessarily have a Machiavellian intent. More likely, naïveté on the administrator's part, regarding the psychologist's necessary role in testing and the psychologist's knowledge of the limitations associated with automated testing, is the culprit.

Marketplace Realities

Given managed care's manifold impact, psychological testing procedures are not conducted today as a "standard order" by the attending psychiatrist or primary therapist within a facility. In some instances, funding for psychological testing may not be available (i.e., it may not be a covered benefit) when it is nevertheless clinically indicated (see Chapter 1). The funding gap is typically dealt with in one of the following ways:

1. No testing is completed.
2. Testing is completed but the psychologist is not paid for it.
3. Testing is completed by a student or an intern under supervision (and the psychologist probably is not paid for the supervision).

As managed care models evolve to all-inclusive services and capitation, psychological testing will be calculated in the monthly premium, because a proportion of patients will always need this service.

The solutions for facility administrators are varied. One possibility would be to hire a testing psychologist, as an employee or as a consultant, to conduct testing where indicated. Few facilities would need a psychologist to conduct testing on a full-time basis. In such circumstances, the psychologist may wish to have more "employability appeal" by providing to the facility other services for which he or she is appropriately trained: individual, group, and family therapy; outcome studies; consultation services; training and in-services, and so on.

At the opposite end of the continuum, a facility's administration may wish to use technology and computerized testing as a solution to operating cost-effectively within all-inclusive or capitated managed care contracts. This solution could be conducted internally within the facility or subcontracted to a technologically sophisticated testing psychologist or practice group. Psychologists wishing to pursue this market must keep a balanced perspective on maintaining high quality while producing reports rapidly and remaining sensitive to the need to keep costs low and competitive. As the market consolidates, costs will undoubtedly be driven even further downward. Practitioners should aim to be efficient, expeditious, and economical. Quality at too high a cost cannot be afforded; thus, its benefit becomes unattainable.

Employee Selection

Testing psychologists have long consulted with industry and corporations in providing employee-candidate screenings. In consideration of the rigors typically associated with the treatment of challenging psychiatric or behaviorally disturbed patients, treatment facilities may wish to use testing psychologists to screen employment applicants for traits that may not bode well in such treatment settings.

The MMPI-2, the 16PF, or various other standard objective tests that have a track record in either employee screening or generalizable norms, are likely the best tools. Hilson Research, Inc. specializes in a variety of objective employee-screening instruments. (Hilson may be contacted at 718-805-0063.) Any procedures adopted should be matched against all legal and regulatory guidelines, to avoid any risks associated with violation of privacy or charges of discrimination. Consultation with an attorney who specializes in labor law is also a well-considered recommendation. Most facilities are expected to adequately screen their staff and are responsible for ensuring patients' and co-workers' safety. Such expectations sometimes place facility administrators and human resource specialists in a difficult position. Testing psychologists, with appropriate training and competence in employee selection measures and processes, will be able to provide much needed assistance.

JCAHO Standards and Psychology

Rarely will a psychologist be conversant with issues involving the Joint Commission on Accreditation of Healthcare Organizations' (JCAHO, 1991). But these issues are important to the operation of any facility wishing to obtain or maintain accreditation status. Rarer still would be a testing psychologist who is aware of the JCAHO standards and requirements. Many facilities rely on JCAHO accreditation as a key to gaining admission to various managed care organizations' provider panels. Thus, for many facilities, JCAHO is the pivotal body in the ability to operate and to gain contracts. Historically, psychologists have had little contact with JCAHO standards. Today, this situation is changing, especially in psychiatric facilities.

Evolving JCAHO standards for initial patient assessment activities are moving away from segregated, discrete, and multiple assessments. Such procedures create frustration for the patient and increase costs for facilities because of the time wasted in such redundant activities. Zappia and Watrons (1995, p. 13) created a flowchart to illustrate such a decision (see Figure 4.3).

Following a detailed examination by a team headed by Zappia and Watrons, the markedly improved and streamlined model shown in Figure 4.4 resulted (p. 14).

The model shows the efficiencies that can be achieved with improved data flow. This model also indicates savings in cost and time, decreased redundancy, better patient response/cooperation with assessments actually conducted, and more expeditious use of everyone's time. Psychologists who are well trained in assessment can add their expertise to procedural design issues that are assessment-related. Psychologists need to begin to think in these broader meta-assessment/design ways.

JCAHO is moving toward ever-increasing emphasis on outcomes and patient satisfaction. These issues are of equal concern to facilities'

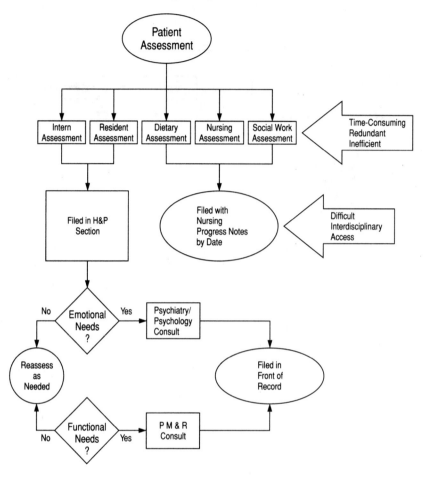

FIGURE 4.3

Current Initial Inpatient Assessment Process

Source: Adapted from "Designing an Integrated, Initial Patient Assessment" by Pat Zappia and Julie Watrons. *Joint Commission Perspectives, 15*(1), p. 13. Copyright © 1995, Joint Commission on Accreditation of Healthcare Organizations. Reprinted with permission.

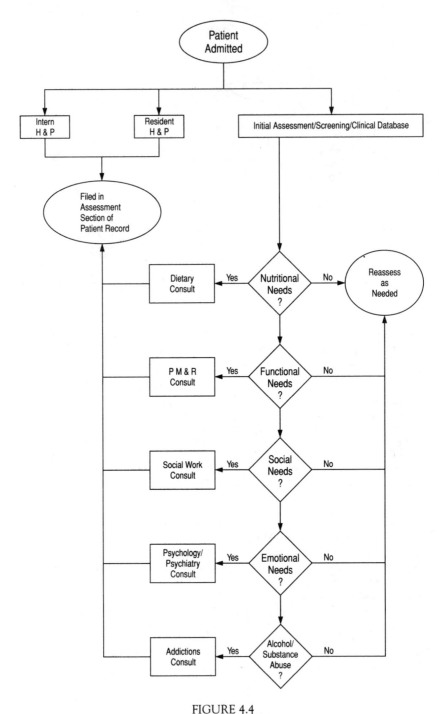

FIGURE 4.4
Proposed Initial Inpatient Assessment Process
Source: Adapted from "Designing an Integrated, Initial Patient Assessment" by Pat Zappia and Julie Watrons. *Joint Commission Perspectives, 15*(1), p. 14. Copyright © 1995, Joint Commission on Accreditation of Healthcare Organizations. Reprinted with permission.

operations. Descriptions and examples will appear in later chapters that focus on outcomes management and quality management.

Conclusion

Testing psychologists who expand their repertoire to include the additional skills outlined in this chapter will be quite well positioned to work, partner, or collaborate with facility administrators in the provision of an improved quality of patient care, an expanded spectrum of patient services, more cost-efficient operations and procedures, and mutually equitable opportunity for the improved profitability of the facility and the practitioner. Not all testing psychologists may wish or be able to pursue facility opportunities; conversely, not all facilities may hold a need for such services. However, for those instances where there is a good fit, there will likely be keen innovation and improved quality of patient care, along with concomitant improvement in the facility's functioning and efficiency.

APPLICATIONS AND BENEFITS OF PSYCHOLOGICAL ASSESSMENT IN A MANAGED CARE SYSTEM

CHAPTER 5

Clinical Outcomes Management

A S THE BEHAVIORAL HEALTHCARE market becomes more consolidated, there will be less variation in fees, and other factors of provider selection will become more influential. In this author's opinion, this is a positive trend for providers, as well as patients, because eventual incentives of differentially higher reimbursement rates and more coveted contracts will go to more skilled therapists. Primary factors in the selection processes will be measured outcomes and clinical efficacy. The caveat attached to this benefit is that the more skilled therapists must be able to *demonstrate* their skills. Testing psychologists may find that their expertise in psychometrics will heighten the demand for their services because clinicians (of all disciplines), facilities, third-party payors, and managed care companies will need guidance in instrument selection and assessment procedures to develop outcomes management systems.

Psychology's Key Role

Psychologists hold a unique and valuable position within behavioral healthcare. They are the only behavioral health professionals systematically trained in psychometrics, research design, and psychological testing techniques. These skills can be brought to bear in designing everything from treatment plans to new models of care. Testing psychologists are well positioned to be drivers of this important added value in behavioral healthcare.

Few practices, facilities, or managed care companies are currently conducting integrated, systemwide, organized investigations. However, in a recent study reported in *Psychotherapy Finances* (Fee, Practice, and Managed Care Survey, 1995, January) 88% of the managed care organizations surveyed stated that "provider selection and other contracting decisions" (p. 1) would be based on outcome data in the future.

The Goal of Standardization: Various Models

There seems to be little current consensus as to what comprises a standard in outcomes measurement. Technological advances and new care delivery models will aid in the development of outcome standards. In addition, active task forces are addressing the following issues (Behavioral Outcomes, 1994, p. 16):

1. Which outcomes to measure, based on an evaluation of existing instruments and the development of new indicators.
2. What standards of data collection to use to ensure accurate, affordable, and practical measures.
3. How to analyze and disseminate information to everyday practice settings in the public and private sector.

For more information on these task forces, the Outcomes Conference, in Washington, DC, may be contacted by calling 202-883-4820.

AMBHA'S REPORT CARD

The American Managed Behavioral Healthcare Association (AMBHA), chaired by Ronald Geraty, M.D. (Executive Vice President of MEDCO Behavioral Healthcare Corporation), is developing a "Report Card" (more on this in Chapter 6) on practice services and care delivery that is quite consumer- and patient-focused (Grinfeld, 1995). These categories are expected to be examined in their report card:

1. Patient Satisfaction.
2. Consumer Assessment of Service Quality.
3. Functional Outcome (Health Status).
4. Accessibility.

AMBHA also notes that there is no current consensus on measures yet, but the fact that categories are selected is a progressive step. Eventually, linkage of such information to medical cost offset will likely be the norm. (See Chapter 8 for more on the current status of medical cost offset.)

MEDICAL OUTCOMES STUDY

Greenfield (1993, p. 432) provides a model of a conceptual framework for outcomes assessment, which appeared in the well-known Medical Outcomes Study (MOS). It has been adapted for behavioral healthcare and appears here as Table 5.1. Because it provides practice pathways for integrated assessment within a seamless design, the model is a practical and cost-effective representation of clinical operations and patient care.

CLINICAL OUTCOMES MANAGEMENT

Ellwood, Huber, and Couch (1991) describe the key criteria for a sound clinical outcome system (p. 468). It must:

1. Measure a patient's functional status and quality of life over time, using terms that are readily understandable by patients and providers.
2. Document changes in a patient's clinical condition over time, as a result of therapy.
3. Ensure that data are collected in a common format, using widely accepted public-domain protocols across a large number of sites.

TABLE 5.1
Conceptual Frameworks for Behavioral Healthcare (Adapted from Greenfield's Medical Outcomes Study, 1993)

Structure of Care	Process of Care	Outcomes
System Characteristics	**Technical Style**	**Clinical End Points**
Organization	Visits	Symptom level reduction
Specialty mix	Medications	
Financial incentive	Referrals	**Functional Status**
Workload	Psychological testing	Physical/Mental/Social/Role
Access/Convenience	Hospitalizations	
	Expenditures	**General Well-Being**
Provider Characteristics	Continuity of care	Health perceptions
Age		Energy/Fatigue
Gender	**Interpersonal Style**	Pain
Ethnicity	Interpersonal manner	Life satisfaction
Specialty training	Patient participation	
Theoretical orientation	Counseling	**Satisfaction with Care**
Economic incentives	Communication level	Access
Beliefs/Attitudes		Conveniences
Preferences		Financial coverage
Job Satisfaction		Quality
		General
Patient Characteristics		
Age		
Gender		
Ethnicity		
Diagnosis/condition		
Severity		
Co-morbid conditions		
Health habits		
Beliefs/Attitudes		
Preferences		

4. Maintain data collected from multiple sites in a single repository, allowing comparisons of patient outcomes.
5. Incorporate standardized and valid methods of accounting for healthcare organizations' effects on health and quality of life.

Testing psychologists are currently in a position to offer marked assistance in designing these systems.

Continuum Model of Service

With the advent of managed care, a variety of adaptations and paradigm shifts have impacted the behavioral healthcare field. Models are being borrowed from public education and schools; the "least restrictive environment" concept is an example. An appropriate level of care is being provided for patients. What is now evolving in clinical behavioral healthcare practice is a continuum of care model. Within the continuum concept, several types of preventive models are developing in HMO and capitated plans, along with new innovative types of outpatient programs. These blend easily into partial hospitalization, day or evening treatment, and weekend programs. Inpatient care is becoming briefer and more intensive, and crisis intervention is more focused. Residential care is rendered for shorter lengths of stay, and independent living and halfway houses are becoming more prevalent.

INTEGRATED OUTCOMES

The role of psychological testing will vary within these models, based on patients' needs. Seamless outcomes management systems will need to be integrated into the new behavioral healthcare continuum. To achieve this integration, outcomes measurement tools need to be concomitant with treatment, not just an ex post facto addition.

Outcomes Management

The basic procedural components of an outcomes management system include:

1. Treatment outcome and functionality.
2. Treatment follow-up.
3. Patient satisfaction.

As additional subcategories, there may also be measures of:

1. A patient's quality of life or level of (nonpsychiatric) functioning.
2. Managed care organization satisfaction.
3. Clinician satisfaction.
4. Cost-for-care data.

INFORMED CONSENT

A prerequisite of any outcome study is a basic informed consent from the client. Regardless of treatment setting, an informed consent is mandatory. Some facilities may require approval from an Institutional Review Board, Research Committee, or Protection of Human Subjects Committee prior to the instigation of any research. Constructing an appropriate informed consent form is a straightforward task (see Figure 5.1).

MEASURING DECISIONS

Before a decision is made to initiate an outcomes management system, a variety of options can be investigated to see what can be measured or how measurements can be conducted. For example, one choice would be to measure across venues of care; the outcomes management system would examine an *episode* of care—from the point of initial contact through discharge. Whether the patient is initially placed in or moves through an inpatient, outpatient, or partial hospitalization treatment setting, the focus is not *where* the patient is treated, but "What was the outcome for treating this specific problem?"

Another model focuses on a variety of diagnoses or sites of care. Examples would be examination of the outcome of depressed patients in an inpatient setting, or how well anxiety-diagnosed patients improve in an outpatient setting. This type of study could focus on the outcome of specific types of diagnostic groups, even though they may be treated in a variety of settings.

102

Clinical Outcomes Management

(Your Letterhead)

INFORMED CONSENT FORM

NAME (print): _____ CLIENT I.D.#: _____ DATE OF BIRTH: ____/____/____

- I hereby consent to being involved in the XYZ Survey, ABC Study, and etc.

- I understand that I will not be identified by name or in any report or summary of this project.

- I understand that I may withdraw consent and discontinue participation in this project at any time and that this will have no bearing on my status in my treatment.

- I understand that I may decline participation in this project and that doing such will not be cause to deny or alter any indicated services to me.

- I understand the procedures of this study meet the regulatory standards set forth by the U.S. Department of Health and Human Service Regulations concerning the protection of participants.

- I understand there are no medical tests or physical procedures. All I will be asked to do is complete x surveys which deal with my opinions, feelings, or experiences and have no right or wrong answers.

- I understand that I and the practitioner can expect the following benefits:
  (a) Improved treatment at "ABC" clinic.
  (b) Addition to general knowledge of behavioral health care.

- If I have any questions about this survey, I can contact Dr. _____ (123-456-7890).

- _____   _____
  (Client's Signature)   (Date)

- _____   _____
  (Parent's or Guardian's Signature) (Date)

- _____   _____
  (Witness' Signature & Printed Name) (Date)

- Signatures required: Adult client (18 or over) and witness: Parent (or guardian) and child plus witness, if child is 12 through 17; Parent (or guardian) and witness, if child is under 12 or patient adjudicated incompetent. [Check with your state's laws concerning ages of signitories.]

Original—Client Chart   Copy—Client

FIGURE 5.1
Sample Informed Consent Form

TREATMENT OUTCOME

There are a number of different types of treatment outcome studies. However, most methodologies can be reduced to the rather straight-forward procedure of pre- and posttreatment testing, where testing typically consists of one or two measures. Regardless of the site of testing (e.g., inpatient, outpatient, or residential), most instruments considered for use should be of short duration and self-administered, and they should lend themselves to quick hand-scoring or computer scanning.

INSTRUMENT SELECTION

Instruments such as the MMPI-2 or California Personality Inventory (CPI) may not be appropriate because of the time it takes a patient to complete them and because, given the shorter lengths of inpatient stay, these tests are not appropriate for pre- and posttreatment measures. When utilized in longer-term settings, such as extended outpatient care consisting of more than 20 to 30 sessions (or greater than 9 months' duration of care) or a residential setting where individuals might be treated for a period longer than 6 months, these instruments may have value.

In most treatment settings, testing psychologists would probably consider the Brief Symptom Inventory (BSI; Derogatis, 1994), the Symptom Check List-90-Revised (SCL-90-R; Derogatis, 1977), or the BASIS-32 (Eisen, Grob, & Klein, 1986). As a general rule, the fewer the number of items on an instrument, the greater the likelihood of user compliance and, presumably, better data. The fact that these instruments are well respected and psychometrically sound makes them top choices for treatment outcomes testing. Additionally, they provide very good data that are beneficial toward treatment planning.

CLINICIAN'S PERSPECTIVE

The SCL-90-Analogue, a very brief companion instrument to the SCL-90-R/BSI, allows the clinician to rank the level of a patient's disturbance. This ranking can act as a beneficial double-check for diagnostic accuracy and perception on the clinician's part. In clinical training programs where diagnostics are involved, it can also be useful as an additional validational measure between a student clinician's perspective of the patient and the patient's own self-report. Equal opportunity for distortion exists in both the clinician's perspective and the patient's viewpoint. However, the utilization of the SCL-90-Analogue in tandem with the patient's self-administered SCL-90-R provides a more robust clinical picture. Similar instruments—for example, the Brief Psychiatric Rating Scale (BPRS; Edell, Joy, & Yehuda, 1990) and the Global Assessment of Functioning (GAF; APA, 1994)—offer additional measures from the clinician's perspective.

Managed care companies or other clinical reviewers may wish to utilize such tools as a means to evaluate a clinician's diagnostic accuracy and appropriate utilization of diagnostic categories. Stout (1993) found that clinicians frequently use Major Depression as a catchall diagnostic category. Use of clinician ratings of patients, in tandem with patient self-reports, should help eliminate overdiagnosis in certain categories.

COLLECTING PATIENT DATA

Although broad-scale data collection is critical for meaningful outcome tracking, it should be a standard practice to obtain informed consent from the patient. If the patient declines participation in the study, then no type of data collection can be sampled with that patient.

In outpatient clinics, one may wish to have the patient come to the office site a half-hour early for the first session, in order to complete initial pretreatment measures prior to starting the session. The instrument should be completed by the client under proctored supervision and NEVER allowed to be taken home to be completed. A general rule of thumb, from this author's experience, is that an outcome instrument that contains more than 100 items should not be used in a treatment setting that is 6 months or shorter in duration.

A percentage of outpatients will move toward a planned termination session and then fail to come to the last session. For this reason, it is wise to administer posttreatment measures at the third- or second-to-the-last scheduled session. In inpatient or residential settings (or any type of setting where the individual stays 24 hours per day), the instrument should be administered within the first 24 to 48 hours of admission and within the last 24 to 48 hours prior to the scheduled discharge.

PRE- AND POSTTREATMENT ASSESSMENT METHODOLOGY

Some researchers (e.g., Kerlinger, 1973) note an inherent weakness of the pre- and posttreatment design: poor control of independent variables. Other factors that are external to the treatment process could influence the results of the testing. In addition, statistically, the regression toward the mean can be problematic for accurate

TABLE 5.2
Comparison of Two Health Evaluation Instruments

Product	Format	Cost	Source
Health Status Questionnaire (HSQ) 2.0	Paper and pencil Computerized	$1.00 each (500 minimum)	National Computer Systems, Inc. 5605 Green Circle Drive Minnetonka, MN 55343 800-627-7271
(Medical Outcome Study) Short Form 36 (SF-36)	Self-administered Interview structure (trained inter- viewer)	$1.00 licensing fee	Ware, J. (1993). *SF-36 Health survey: Manual & intro- duction guide.* Boston: Nimrod Press.

interpretation of results. Such issues are important scientifically, but the realities of managed care would dictate that "half a loaf" must be perceived as better than none. However, when reporting outcome results externally, clinicians and facilities measuring outcomes should keep those confounding factors in mind, and draw attention to them.

The level of technology involved is at the discretion of the tester. Most of the instruments discussed thus far are available in hand-scorable formats (which do not take a great deal of time) as well as computer-scorable formats. If a high-volume outcome assessment is undertaken, it may be most cost-effective to use computer-scored versions. Another alternative is to utilize and appropriately train paraprofessionals or graduate students to hand-score these instruments. Interpretation remains solely the psychologist's domain. Detailed information on these and other measures is listed in the Appendix.

Capabilities	Advantages	Disadvantages
Measure general level of functioning, well-being, perception of overall health Medical and psychiatric population	Eight health attributes Index of health status change 14 years and older Level of functioning instrument Outcome instrument	Not appropriate for child populations Little focus on psychiatric issues per se
Various health concept measurements: • Physical activity limitation • Usual role limitation • General mental health • General health perception • Social activity limitation • Pain • Emotional problem	Good reliability Good validity Brief Machine-scored	Not appropriate for child populations Little focus on psychiatric issues per se

FUNCTIONAL STATUS

The outcomes management area of functional status is currently widening its focus and increasing in popularity. However, patient functionality is a term used in a variety of ways. In some instances, this concept is thought to refer to DSM Axis V types of functioning and ratings. There are pros and cons to this practice. The benefits are that it is a widely accepted measure well known by all, and it is fairly standardized in *DSM-IV*. However, a problem arises in that Axis V is not a patient self-report; it is a clinician report. In the early stages of treatment, the clinician may not be able to provide the most accurate data.

In response to these shortcomings, supplemental information may help. One way to achieve this is by utilizing instruments that measure more general levels of functioning, such as the Health Status Questionnaire, version 2.0 (HSQ 2.0) or the Short Form 36 (SF 36). These instruments, which are further described in Table 5.2 on pages 106–107, are variations of one concept. They provide an overall evaluation of health (health perception from the patient's perspective). Some individuals and sites have developed their own (less empirically validated) instruments to examine various functional status issues of employment, recidivism, continuing care, contentment, and so on. (These types of instruments are discussed in the next section, "Treatment Follow-Up.")

The National Association of Psychiatric Health Systems (NAPHS, formerly the National Association of Private Psychiatric Hospitals) has a "Graphic Model" and methodology that examines various levels of outcome/status on these parameters:

1. Physical Mobility.
2. Personal Treatment Needs.
3. Treatment Consumption.
4. Self-Concept, Concept of Others.
5. Social Mobility.
6. Shelter Needs.
7. Economic Consumption.

These parameters help to, first, determine an individual's treatment needs, and, second, reflect the client's progress or the intervention's outcome. The model can be obtained from NAPHS by calling 202-393-6700. Additional evaluation instruments are noted in Tables 5.3 and 5.4.

Treatment Follow-Up

Treatment follow-up differs from patient outcome in that treatment follow-up is a measure of how well treatment has impacted on the

TABLE 5.3
"All -Purpose" Scales

Product	Source
Denver Community Mental Health Questionnaire (DCMHQ): • *Multidimensional measure, 79 items* • *Social functioning measure* • *Specific symptomatology report*	Ciarlo, J., & Reihman, J. (1977). Development of a multi-dimensional program evaluation instrument. In R. Coursey, G. Spector, S. Murrell, & B. Hunt (Eds.), *Program evaluation for mental health: Methods, strategies, and participants* (pp. 131–167). New York: Grune and Stratton.
Major Problem Rating System: • *Self-report* • *Computerized format* • *280 items* • *Outcome measurement (assessed only in areas identified as problems by respondents)* • *44 categories of functioning* • *Social functioning measure* • *Specific symptomatology report*	Stevenson, J., McCullough, L., Stout, R., & Longabaugh, R. (1989). The development of an individualized, problem-oriented psychiatric outcome measure. *Evaluation & The Health Professions, 12(2),* 134–158.
Target Complaints: • *Problem severity/improvement measure* • *Social functioning measure* • *Specific symptomatology report*	Battle, C., Imber, S., Hoehn-Saric, R., & Stark, J. (1966). Target complaints as criteria of improvement. *American Journal of Psychotherapy, 20,* 184–192.

TABLE 5.4
Integrated Agency and Service Instruments

Product	Format	Source
Child and Adolescent Services Assessment (CASA) **Child and Adolescent Psychiatry Assessment (CAPA)**	Interview structure (20 minutes) Children and parents are informants	Angold, A. (1991). *The Child and Adolescent Psychiatric Assessment, version 2.1* (3 months). Durham, NC: Duke University Medical Center. *or* Burns, B. (1991). *Child and Adolescent Services Assessment, version 3.0.* Durham, NC: Duke University Medical Center.
Child and Youth Services Agency Network Survey (CYSANS)	Self-administered questionnaire (mailed survey) Five-point Likert Scale	Morrisey, J. P. (1992). An interorganizational network approach to evaluating children's mental health services systems. In L. Bickman & D. J. Rog (Eds.), *Evaluating mental health services for children.* San Francisco: Jossey-Bass.

Capabilities	Advantages	Disadvantages
Links mental health problems to service use Expanded list of child-specific services across multiple service sectors Parent/Family service related to child's emotional/behavioral problem Link between setting/provider type/source of reimbursement Family burden assessment Used in conjunction with Child and Adolescent Assessment (CAPA)	Service use benefits investigation Single day of interviewer training	
Linkage information (network agency organizations): • Other agency awareness • Community policy/ program influence • Client referrals • Funds exchanges • Information flows • Intra-agency communication flow • Agency coordination • Agency helpfulness measures • Relationship satisfaction • Disagreement measurement	Global, integrated instrument	Limited to youth services agencies

patient's life during x number of months after completion of care or discharge (e.g., 6 months after discharge from inpatient treatment or 12 months after completion of outpatient care).

FREQUENCY OF DATA COLLECTION AND INSTRUMENTATION

There must be a basic determination of how often data are to be collected. The general rules of thumb are 6, 12, and 24 months, or 3, 12, and 18 months after completion of treatment. Clinician-researchers must realize that, in some instances, treatment may be ongoing and concomitant; that is, a patient may be discharged from inpatient care and 6 months later he or she may still be involved in outpatient aftercare. Or, someone may be rehospitalized and again involved in inpatient care. Any instruments that are utilized in treatment follow-up should be sensitive to these types of possibilities.

One appealing option for assessing treatment follow-up is to employ the same instrument that was used at intake and discharge. This approach provides consistency of measures over time. Alternatively, the user may wish to develop his or her own specific instrument and tools. An example of an instrument developed by this author appears in Figure 5.2. It was specifically tailored to address a variety of issues that were of concern to an inpatient facility, based on follow-up findings on discharged inpatients. Such instruments are often more like data collection tools and questionnaires than clinical instruments. They are typically composed of a variety of numeric check-offs, Likert Scales, and/or comment sections that can be remarkably helpful and useful in the clinical management and clinical administrative processes.

FOLLOW-UP ASSESSMENT METHODOLOGY

Follow-up assessments should be administered on a set schedule at predetermined interval points. In one approach, the instrument is mailed to former patients with a self-addressed, stamped return envelope, and a cover letter requesting the discharged patient's participation.

ABC Hospital Treatment Follow-Up Project
Adult Survey—IV

Name: _____ Sex: _____ 1. M _____ 2. F

Unit: _____ Physician _____

Diagnosis on admission _____

Diagnosis on discharge _____

Length of stay _____ days   Number previous hosp. _____
     Interval: _____ 1. 3 months

Respondent: _____   _____ 2. 6 months
     _____ 3. 9 months

ID#: _____ Age: _____   _____ 4. 12 months

Marital status: _____ 1. Married _____ 2. Divorced _____
     3. Widowed _____ 4. Co-habit _____
     5. Single _____

1. Current residence
    _____ a self
    _____ b. spouse/mate
    _____ c. family
    _____ d. friend(s)
    _____ e. residential facility
    _____ f. halfway house
    _____ g. other _____

2. Current work status
    _____ a. full-time
    _____ b. part-time
    _____ c. none
    _____ d. retired

3. If working, have you been working steadily?
    _____ a. yes
    _____ b. no

4. If not working, any work since discharge?
    _____ a. yes
    _____ b. no

5. Describe adjustment to work
    _____ a. excellent
    _____ b. good
    _____ c. fair
    _____ d. poor   *(continued)*

FIGURE 5.2
Sample Treatment Follow-Up Survey: Adult Version

6. Currently in school?

_____ a. yes
_____ b. no

7. Describe adjustment to school

_____ a. excellent
_____ b. good
_____ c. fair
_____ d. poor

8. Estimate overall improvement during hospitalization

_____ a. excellent
_____ b. good
_____ c. fair
_____ d. poor
_____ e. not apply

9. Overall condition now

_____ a. excellent
_____ b. good
_____ c. fair
_____ d. poor

10. Reason for discharge

_____ a. attainment of treatment goals
_____ b. financial reasons
_____ c. transfer
_____ d. family decision
_____ e. staff person
_____ f. self

11. Condition on discharge

_____ a. recovered
_____ b. significant improvement
_____ c. moderate improvement
_____ d. mild improvement
_____ e. unchanged
_____ f. worse

12. Treatment after hospitalization

_____ a. back to prior outpatient therapist
_____ b. continued to see same therapist as inpatient
_____ c. referred to social service agency
_____ d. none
_____ e. in-house referral to outpatient therapist
_____ f. other _____

FIGURE 5.2 (Continued)

13. Type of treatment
    _____ a. individual
    _____ b. family
    _____ c. group
    _____ d. spouse/marital

14. Is treatment continuing at this time?
    _____ a. by whom _____
    _____ b. type _____
    _____ c. no

15. Currently on any medications?
    _____ a. yes
    _____ b. no

16. Type of medication
    _____ a. antidepressant _____
    _____ b. antipsychotic _____
    _____ c. antimanic _____
    _____ d. anxiolytic _____
    _____ e. stimulant _____
    _____ f. other _____

17. Rehospitalization since ABC?
    _____ a. yes
    _____ b. no

18. Was hospitalization for same problem?
    _____ a. yes
    _____ b. no

19. Condition now, compared to condition at discharge
    _____ a. marked improvement
    _____ b. some improvement
    _____ c. maintained
    _____ d. declined

20. Management now of problems experienced before hospitalization
    _____ a. excellent
    _____ b. good
    _____ c. fair
    _____ d. poor

21. Relationship with family
    _____ a. excellent
    _____ b. good
    _____ c. fair
    _____ d. poor

FIGURE 5.2 (Continued)

22. Relationship with spouse
       _____ a. excellent
       _____ b. good
       _____ c. fair
       _____ d. poor

23. Relationship with peers
       _____ a. excellent
       _____ b. good
       _____ c. fair
       _____ d. poor

24. Describe thinking processes
       _____ a. excellent
       _____ b. good
       _____ c. fair
       _____ d. poor

25. Describe social interaction
       _____ a. excellent
       _____ b. good
       _____ c. fair
       _____ d. poor

26. Mood
       _____ a. excellent
       _____ b. good
       _____ c. fair
       _____ d. poor

27. Sleeping pattern
       _____ a. excellent
       _____ b. good
       _____ c. fair
       _____ d. poor

28. Any alcohol abuse?
       _____ a. yes
       _____ b. no

28a. If yes, what type?
       _____ beer
       _____ hard liquor
       _____ wine/coolers

28b. If yes, how often?
       _____ daily
       _____ 2–3 times/week
       _____ 2–3 times/month

FIGURE 5.2 (Continued)

29. Any drug abuse?

_____ a. yes
_____ b. no

29a. If yes, what type?

_____ pot/hash
_____ opiates
_____ heroin
_____ cocaine/crack
_____ uppers (speed, amphetamines)
_____ downers (quaaludes, valium)

29b. If yes, how often (over all)?

_____ daily
_____ 2–3 times/week
_____ 2–3 times/month

30. Hospital care

_____ a. excellent
_____ b. good
_____ c. fair
_____ d. poor

31. Psychiatrist's care

_____ a. excellent
_____ b. good
_____ c. fair
_____ d. poor

32. Communication with psychiatrist

_____ a. excellent
_____ b. good
_____ c. fair
_____ d. poor

33. Was there a psychologist, social worker, or certified addiction counselor involved in treatment?

_____ a. yes (name) _____
_____ b. no

34. Psychologist care

_____ a. excellent
_____ b. good
_____ c. fair
_____ d. poor

35. Social worker care

_____ a. excellent
_____ b. good
_____ c. fair
_____ d. poor

FIGURE 5.2 (Continued)

36. Certified addiction counselor care
    _____ a. excellent
    _____ b. good
    _____ c. fair
    _____ d. poor

37. Nursing/Psych tech care
    _____ a. excellent
    _____ b. good
    _____ c. fair
    _____ d. poor

38. Costs covered by insurance
    _____ a. all
    _____ b. most
    _____ c. some
    _____ d. none

39. Expected costs of hospitalization
    _____ a. lower than expected
    _____ b. expected
    _____ c. higher than expected
    _____ d. no idea of costs

40. If you had to do it over, would you seek admission at ABC Hospital?
    _____ a. yes
    _____ b. no

41. Would you recommend ABC Hospital?
    _____ a. yes
    _____ b. no

42. What was the most important factor in your recovery?
    _____ a. hospitalization
    _____ b. therapy/outpatient
    _____ c. family support
    _____ d. other _____

43. How have you adjusted to life outside of the hospital since discharge?
    _____ a. difficulty readjusting
    _____ b. moderate difficulty readjusting
    _____ c. easy adjustment

44. How stressful has your life been postdischarge?
    _____ a. very stressful
    _____ b. moderately stressful
    _____ c. no difference
    _____ d. little stress/less stressful

FIGURE 5.2 (Continued)

118

45. What did you like best about ABC Hospital?

_____

_____

_____

46. What didn't you like about ABC Hospital?

_____

_____

_____

47. What type(s) of therapy helped most?

_____

_____

_____

_____

48. Any additional comments

_____

_____

_____

FIGURE 5.2 (Continued)

(Informed consent would have been gained at the beginning of care, perhaps in tandem with the treatment outcome agreement.) In this author's experience, return rates within some inpatient populations (perhaps also with other populations) have been relatively poor. A preferred methodology has been to involve appropriately trained paraprofessionals in data collection via telephone calls. These individuals must be thoroughly instructed about issues of confidentiality and informed about psychopathology. Upon follow-up, some former patients will be discovered to need continued clinical care or a renewal of psychotherapeutic services. It is important to have research staff who can refer the individual back to the initial treating clinician or to an appropriate emergency room or crisis line.

Although, ideally, each patient would be contacted after discharge, if the client base is large, this goal can be impractical. As a substitute, random sampling can suffice. It is recommended that at least one out of three or one out of five discharged patients be contacted.

The technology necessary to deploy follow-up outcomes assessment consists of a computerized database to track results and a statistical package for data analysis. Staffing would be comprised of a variety of appropriately trained staff and/or volunteers. Costs vary as a function of instruments purchased and the time required to collect the data. Additional costs can be incurred even when using one's own instruments, because of the time needed for data entry, subsequent statistical analysis, and report production. (The total would vary as a function of the labor costs associated with such procedures.)

Patient Satisfaction

INSTRUMENTATION

Patient satisfaction surveys have become quite popular in many clinical circumstances (see Chapter 6). In this author's opinion, patient satisfaction instruments are best developed by individuals who will be using the findings. Psychometric rigor should not be ignored in such surveys. Safeguards against skewed results must be in place, and the surveys should utilize questions that get at negative issues (e.g., "What didn't you like . . . ?") as well as general or positive considerations. Provision of even number rankings (e.g., 1–4, 1–6) and avoidance of "middle-of-the-road" options (by using quasi-forced choice) are also important. A sample of a patient satisfaction survey used and developed by this author appears in Figure 5.3. Larsen et al. (1979) developed a standardized tool for client satisfaction. Its features are summarized in Table 5.5. The Mental Health Corporation of America has also developed a satisfaction measurement system that is gaining use.

One of the best methods for instrumentation development is to examine a variety of different types of patient satisfaction surveys

Clinical Outcomes Management

The quality of care provided by ABC Hospital is evaluated on an ongoing basis. We therefore ask that you take a few moments to tell us how we can improve. Your opinion will help us know how we may best serve our patients and community. Thank you for your time and consideration.

Completed by: Patient _____   Parent _____   Guardian _____

Date completed: _____/_____/_____ Unit name: _____ House case: Yes/No

Staff responsible for completion _____

How did you hear about our facility?   _____

_____ 1. Present psychiatrist	_____ 9. Courts/probation
_____ 2. Family physician	officer/police
_____ 3. Family	_____ 10. TV ad
_____ 4. Friend	_____ 11. Radio ad
_____ 5. Psychologist	_____ 12. Paper/magazine ad
_____ 6. Social worker	_____ 13. Insurance company
_____ 7. Addictions counselor	_____ 14. Crisis line
_____ 8. School personnel	_____ 15. Other _____

How would you rate the following (Please circle your answer and comment specifically on items rates 3 or 4. Comments on items rated 1 or 2 would be appreciated):

	Strongly Agree	Mildly Agree	Mildly Disagree	Strongly Disagree	Not Applicable
1. ADMISSION OFFICE (admission to the hospital):					
a. The Admission staff member was pleasant and courteous.	1	2	3	4	5
b. The Admissions Officer was helpful in explaining the papers I signed.	1	2	3	4	5
Comments: _____					
2. ADMISSION BY UNIT STAFF (admission to the unit):					
a. During my Admission onto the unit, unit staff treated me with consideration and respect.	1	2	3	4	5
Comments: _____					

(continued)

FIGURE 5.3
Patient Satisfaction Survey

	Strongly Agree	Mildly Agree	Mildly Disagree	Strongly Disagree	Not Applicable
3. QUALITY OF CARE:					
a. The care provided by my psychiatrist was beneficial.	1	2	3	4	5
Comments:					
b. The care provided by my psychologist was beneficial.	1	2	3	4	5
Comments:					
c. The care provided by my certified alcohol counselor was beneficial.	1	2	3	4	5
Comments:					
d. The care provided by my social worker was beneficial.	1	2	3	4	5
Comments:					
4. UNIT STAFF (Nurses and Techs):					
a. The staff was courteous and helpful.	1	2	3	4	5
b. The care was beneficial.	1	2	3	4	5
Comments:					
5. ACTIVITY THERAPY DEPARTMENT (e.g., leisure, education, workshop, teams challenge course):					
a. The staff was courteous and helpful	1	2	3	4	5
b. The care was beneficial.	1	2	3	4	5
Comments:					

FIGURE 5.3 (Continued)

	Strongly Agree	Mildly Agree	Mildly Disagree	Strongly Disagree	Not Applicable
6. TUTORING SERVICES (school; adolescents and children only):					
a. The care was courteous and helpful.	1	2	3	4	5
b. The care was beneficial.	1	2	3	4	5

Comments: _____

7. LAB/X-RAY/EEG/STAFF					
a. The staff was courteous and helpful.	1	2	3	4	5
b. The staff treated me in a professional manner.	1	2	3	4	5

Comments: _____

8. FINANCIAL SERVICES:					
a. The Business Office staff was helpful and efficient in providing assistance in financial matters.	1	2	3	4	5

Comments: _____

9. ACCOMMODATIONS:					
a. The community areas (i.e., dayroom, TV room) were attractive, clean and comfortable	1	2	3	4	5
b. My individual room was attractive, clean and comfortable.	1	2	3	4	5

Comments: _____

FIGURE 5.3 (Continued)

	Strongly Agree	Mildly Agree	Mildly Disagree	Strongly Disagree	Not Applicable
10. FOOD SERVICE:					
a. The food service was of high quality.	1	2	3	4	5
b. The food was served in sufficient quantity.	1	2	3	4	5
c. Dietary staff were courteous.	1	2	3	4	5

Comments: _____

11. DISPOSITIONAL/DISCHARGE PLANNING:

	Strongly Agree	Mildly Agree	Mildly Disagree	Strongly Disagree	Not Applicable
a. If needed, Vocational Counseling was provided and beneficial.	1	2	3	4	5
b. If needed, I was assisted in planning for living arrangements after discharge.	1	2	3	4	5
c. Arrangements were made for follow-up counseling after discharge.	1	2	3	4	5
12. Overall, my stay was beneficial.	1	2	3	4	5

Comments: _____

	Strongly Agree	Mildly Agree	Mildly Disagree	Strongly Disagree	Not Applicable
13. Friends and relatives were treated in a courteous and professional manner when they visited or phoned.	1	2	3	4	5

Comments: _____

14. If a friend needed this facility, I would recommend it. _____

15. What were the most helpful experiences, activities, or therapies during your hospital stay?

_____

FIGURE 5.3 (Continued)

	Strongly Agree	Mildly Agree	Mildly Disagree	Strongly Disagree	Not Applicable
16. What did you dislike about your hospitalization? _____					_____
17. What would you recommend to improve our facility and services? _____					_____
18. Is there any Doctor/Therapist you feel deserves special recognition? _____					_____
19. Is there any employee you feel deserves special recognition? _____					_____
20. General Comments? _____					_____

Thank you for your input.

Please return this survey to staff.
(Staff: Return to Research Mailbox.)

FIGURE 5.3 (Continued)

and measures, and then adapt them into a hybrid that best fits the setting and the users' needs. Considerations fall into at least three areas: (a) technical, (b) clinical, and (c) problematic. If the examinee is a facility, questions should likely deal with:

1. Physical comfort level of the patient's room.
2. Adequacy and quality of the food preparation and delivery.
3. Access to telephones, and access of staff.
4. Availability and courtesy of staff.
5. Opinions of doctors.
6. Convenience.
7. Safety.

TABLE 5.5
Standardized Client Satisfaction Questionnaire

Product	Format	Cost	Source
Client Satisfaction Questionnaire (CSQ-8)	Paper and pencil	Free with permission of author	Attkisson, C., & Zwick, B. (1982). The Client Satisfaction Questionnaire (CSQ-8): Psychometric properties and correlations with service utilization and psychotherapy outcome. *Evaluation and Program Planning, 24,* 233–237.

In an outpatient setting, the instrument may assess:

1. How quickly phone messages are returned.
2. How politely and promptly office staff meet a patients' needs.
3. Whether billing procedures are managed at a satisfactory level (if not, what are the problems?).
4. Whether the office (location) is convenient.
5. Whether parking is available/safe/checked or guarded by security personnel.

The second area of concern would be clinical:

1. Were the patients satisfied with the types, levels, and adequacy of care?
2. Did they find the types of care they received helpful?
3. Would they recommend the facility, the doctor, or the clinic to someone else who was in need of similar types of care?

The final issue is the assessment of problematic areas. This author recommends that specific issues of *dissatisfaction* be reviewed. This approach would include questions assessing:

Capabilities	Advantages	Disadvantages
Eight-item scale High internal consistency General satisfaction measure	Self-administered Rapid completion Rapid scoring	General

1. What types of improvement in care might be made?
2. What areas are weak spots that should be a focus of further development?
3. What was the *least* helpful type of activity that the patient was involved with?
4. If a patient would not be recommending the care administered, why not?

Answers to these and similar questions could be remarkably helpful, although somewhat uncomfortable, for the clinician or administrator to review. Answers can lead to vast improvements in the quality of care, while simultaneously decreasing associated risk issues.

This author also recommends combining numeric responses with opportunity for comment. It is a frustrating experience to uncover interesting numeric data and trends, but to have no supporting comment or information as to why something is well liked and something else is disliked. In such circumstances, comments can be very helpful toward clarifying what a patient's ratings really mean. Use of a Likert Scale with a range of one to four [e.g., Strongly Agree (1), Mildly Agree (2), Mildly Disagree (3), Strongly Disagree (4)] plus Not Applicable creates implicit forced choice of being either pro or con toward the "agree" or "disagree" spectrum. The likelihood of missing data diminishes when the patient can use the Not Applicable response.

PATIENT SATISFACTION ASSESSMENT METHODOLOGY

Ideal methodology and sampling would allow soliciting patients' satisfaction throughout their treatment. For an outpatient, every third session, or a similar schedule, would be helpful. At the very least, patient satisfaction should be solicited as treatment is ending, or just after completion of treatment. Assessment of patient satisfaction at regular intervals may afford opportunities for midcourse correction and continuous quality improvement. Waiting until the patient is finished with treatment, and *then* instituting some type of recommended change, does not benefit that particular patient.

To avoid sampling bias, it is important that every patient have the opportunity to complete a satisfaction survey, regardless of the venue of care. The technology is similar to that of treatment follow-up studies. Data collection via self-administered tools is followed by transcription of the comments and input of the numeric data into a database for compiling statistical analysis and subsequent report productions. Some software programs from NCS, Cardiff, and others provide limited optical character recognition (OCR) capabilities. (See also Chapter 9.)

Additional Satisfaction Evaluations

From a management perspective, it is important that clinicians accept (if not embrace) the idea of patient satisfaction. Some clinicians may be concerned about being evaluated in such a way. Ideally, clinicians should *share* a role in the development of any type of outcome studies methodology that aims to improve the instrument's design and likely decrease clinicians' initial resistances to being evaluated. Most individuals tend to be more involved and engaged when they are "acted with" as opposed to "acted upon."

It is also important to assess and monitor the satisfaction of managed care organizations (MCOs). This assessment should be ongoing and should be conducted with the goal of customer satisfaction, the MCO being the customer. A sample appears in Figure 5.4. Such a survey can provide dramatic feedback that could be pivotal to maintaining one's position in an MCO's network.

Proof of Treatment/Assessment Efficacy

Outcomes management systems have the additional benefit of providing information that may be helpful in marketing services. In this author's opinion, as more and more practices and facilities are placed on an equal playing field with regard to fees, the fourth-party reviewers and third-party payors will become more selective as to provider inclusion based on performance data. Practices and facilities that have a large pool of favorable outcome data to demonstrate the effectiveness of those services will have a definite advantage in winning new contracts.

The point is that psychology needs to examine efficacy. With regard to assessment, psychology needs to be able to develop models that quantify the value (i.e., both cost and benefit) of psychological testing. Within an outcomes management paradigm, psychology can compare the outcomes of cases that had psychological testing conducted and cases that did not. A hypothesis could be that cases for which psychological test batteries (or other types of abbreviated testing) were completed would have an improved treatment outcome as a result of improved diagnostic capabilities. Such patients may have shorter lengths of stay but achieve treatment outcomes equivalent to those realized by patients who had longer lengths of stay but no psychological testing.

Even though it may be distasteful for someone with professional training to seemingly have to justify to a payor the merit and value of his or her work, it is nevertheless the current drive of the marketplace, and psychologists must be prepared to do so. Psychologists are in a special position of being able to have research training in addition to

ABC Systems holds as one of its goals to continually better improve service and value to its customers. It is part of our mission, in fact. As a means to this end, we are very interested in how you perceive our performance. We would appreciate your responses to this survey. It should only take a few minutes of your time. An SASE is enclosed for your convenience. Or you may fax it via 123-456-7890.

If you have any questions, please contact Dr. Chris E. Stout (123-456-7890 x580). Thank you!

	Strongly Agree	Mildly Agree	Mildly Disagree	Strongly Disagree	Not Applicable
1. How would you rate ABC Systems' Case Management Staff:					
a. Timeliness of Review	1	2	3	4	5
Comments:					
b. Quality/Content of Review	1	2	3	4	5
Comments:					
c. Access to Information	1	2	3	4	5
Comments:					
d. Telephone Access	1	2	3	4	5
Comments:					
e. Professionalism	1	2	3	4	5
Comments:					
f. Attitude	1	2	3	4	5
Comments:					
g. Cooperation	1	2	3	4	5
Comments:					
h. Access to Clinicians via UM Staff	1	2	3	4	5
Comments:					

FIGURE 5.4
MCO Satisfaction Survey

Clinical Outcomes Management

	Strongly Agree	Mildly Agree	Mildly Disagree	Strongly Disagree	Not Applicable
2. How helpful is ABC's UM Case Managing in:					
a. Treatment Planning	1	2	3	4	5
Comments: _____					
b. Discharge Planning	1	2	3	4	5
Comments: _____					
c. Continuous Quality Improvement	1	2	3	4	5
Comments: _____					
d. Outcomes	1	2	3	4	5
Comments: _____					
3. How helpful is ABC's Billing/ Accounting Department in:					
a. Timeliness	1	2	3	4	5
Comments: _____					
b. Resolution of Billing Problems	1	2	3	4	5
Comments: _____					
c. Ease of working with staff in Billing problems	1	2	3	4	5
Comments: _____					
d. Ease of working with staff in Adjustment Problems	1	2	3	4	5
Comments: _____					
e. How would you rate the cooperativeness of our Billing Staff?	1	2	3	4	5
Comments: _____					

FIGURE 5.4 (Continued)

4. Are there any staff members you feel deserve special recognition? If so, please note such and state why. _____

_____

5. What problem(s) do you feel are chronic for ABC staff? _____

_____

6. What do you feel ABC does particularly well? _____

_____

7. How could we better serve you in the future? _____

_____

Thank you for your time and assistance!

FIGURE 5.4 (Continued)

clinical training (unlike any other mental health professional). Psychologists are able to conduct studies that are empirically and scientifically rigorous, and to validly demonstrate the utility of their work and the value it provides in improving the quality of clinical care.

Other questions for testing psychologists to consider are:

1. How do you know how good your psychological reports are?
2. What "value added" is a result of your psychological testing?
3. If a patient is/is not provided with psychological testing, what difference does it make in the quality of care or the treatment outcome that this individual will experience?
4. If a psychologist believes that his or her testing provides an important addition to treatment via diagnostic benefit, how should he or she demonstrate it?

To think about assessment and treatment outcome is to think of demonstrating how effective and how beneficial psychological testing is for the patient. When psychologists can empirically demonstrate that psychological testing does provide improved care, then it is incumbent on psychology to be even more specific. For example:

1. How helpful is psychological testing in decreasing treatment cost?
2. Does it decrease other types of additional evaluations, or staff time involved in redundant interviewing?

3. Does a test battery expedite care, making it more efficient and more clinically beneficial?
4. Are psychologists able to tailor their practice to the needs of facilities, clinics, agencies, or payors, as well as patients?

We may find that different sites, different patients, and different payors all have different needs. The referral question is then tailored to the needs of the patient and to other pragmatic and practical considerations.

Outcomes studies are here to stay. They are currently gaining great popularity and notoriety at numerous workshops and seminars, and in reports and books. At this point, psychologists need to enhance the sophistication of the outcome studies models that currently exist. General evolution will occur, but psychologists also need to provide greater emphasis on specific types of outcome issues involving psychological assessment.

A variety of industry collaborations indicate the drive of outcomes studies. Digital Equipment Corporation is involved in three projects evaluating depression treatment efficacy. CNR, a managed care company based in Milwaukee, Wisconsin, is collaborating with the National Institute of Mental Health on outcomes studies. MCC, based in Minnesota, is working with the University of Minnesota on a variety of outcomes studies. Westinghouse and Raytheon are also initiating behavioral health outcomes studies. Charter Hospital Corporation bought an entire outcome study practice a few years ago, and is utilizing that practice's services within all its psychiatric facilities across the country. CPC, National Medical Enterprises, and Columbia/HCA have all initiated similar types of studies within their psychiatric settings.

Conclusion

The purpose of outcomes management is to examine both the clinical and the fiscal features of behavioral healthcare service. Testing psychologists can provide unique assistance in the conceptualization,

TABLE 5.6
Turnkey Automated Systems

Product	Source	Capabilities
Compass System	Compass Information Services, Inc. Radnor Plaza 320 King of Prussia Road Radnor, PA 19087 610-688-2700	Standardized data about patient status Reliable and accurate "snapshot" of patient status over time Treatment progress reports Tracking system that aids in monitoring clinician effectiveness Measure of "return" on dollars spent on outpatient therapy, in terms of improvement the patient experiences (overall, and per session)
Connex MCO	Strategic Decision Systems 5575-B Chamblee Dunwoody Road, Suite 388 Atlanta, GA 30338-4177 800-845-6505	Capitated contract performance Patient satisfaction Patient outcome Contract compliance Costs by CPT code, provider, patient, or period Case management documentation Interface with electronic claims payment Credentials Demographics analysis Claims management Revenue calculation Contract profitability analysis
Connex Provider	Strategic Decision Systems 5575-B Chamblee Dunwoody Road, Suite 388 Atlanta, GA 30338-4177 800-845-6505	Financial performance reporting Contract tracking Recertification documentation Contract profitability calculations Service use monitoring Contract profitability analysis Referral tracking Precertification Referral tracking and rating

TABLE 5.6 (Continued)

Product	Source	Capabilities
Human Service Information System	ECHO Management Group 1055 Taylor Avenue, Suite 300 Baltimore, MD 21286 800-783-7610	Client profiling Scheduling and activity Accounts receivable Management reporting Clinical management Managed care Treatment plans Progress notes Statistical reporting
InStream Provider Network	InStream Corporation 300 Union Park Drive Woburn, MA 01801 617-935-2100	Linkage with providers to MCOs Electronic communications network for productivity tools Intelligent forms Decrease in overhead costs, reduction in data errors and billing omissions "Subscriber" format
Quick Doc—QA	Docutral, Inc. 204 East Joppa Road Penthouse Suite 10 Towson, MD 21286 410-418-8510	Intake reports Progress and SOAP notes Termination summaries Initial treatment plans Treatment plan updates Quality assurance reports Health Status Questionnaire (HSQ) 2.0 Timberland Child Functioning Scale Patient satisfaction questionnaire
Starting Line: System for Outcomes Management	Response Technologies, Inc. 1485 South Country Trail East Greenwich, RI 02818	Quality of life patient profile Patient satisfaction (GHAA Customer Satisfaction) Personal characteristics profile Adult health risk inventory Database management Health Status Profile (SF-36) Basis-32 (add-on module for outcome measurement and symptomatology)

instrumentation, and design of systems. Goals for innovative models would include:

1. Greater specificity of data.
2. Tailoring of methods, procedures, or reports to a specific payor's or facility's needs.
3. Improved, less biased, data-based decision making.
4. Measures of clinical performance and associated costs.
5. Improved triage and referral procedures.
6. Demonstrable quality of care.
7. Ongoing referral tracking with clinical monitoring.
8. Overlay of quality initiatives along with risk management concerns.
9. Feedback mechanisms for data flow and improvement opportunity.
10. Integrated real-time utilization management activities.

Table 5.6 on pages 134–135, provides descriptions of turnkey automated systems currently available. The list is not exhaustive; new developments and improvements are the norm.

CHAPTER 6

Treatment and Quality Management

$\mathcal{Q}$UALITY IMPROVEMENT HAS made remarkable inroads in manufacturing and service industries. It is now making a transition to healthcare, behavioral healthcare, and education. The guiding concepts are referred to as Total Quality Management (TQM), Continuous Quality Improvement (CQI), and other variations on the theme of quality. Historically, medical hospitals had "quality assurance" departments that monitored various aspects of patient care and risk mitigation—after the fact. Today, these departments are known as Quality Management or Quality Improvement Departments, and they take a proactive position within hospitals and facilities. The Joint Commission on Accreditation of Healthcare Organizations (JCAHO) published a booklet, *Transitions from QA to CQI: Using CQI Approaches to Monitor, Evaluate, and Improve Quality* (1991), that is helpful for understanding and operationalizing quality improvement.

The concept of empirically determined and measured quality standards has existed for more than a half century (Shewhart, 1939), but the renewed interest today is attributed to the late W. Edwards Deming, who is considered the originating and driving force behind TQM/CQI. (For purposes of this chapter, the term TQM will be used to represent both concepts.)

Quality Adoption Problems

TQM concepts are currently in vogue at many companies, as evidenced by business schools' consensus and the profusion of management seminars and books on the topic. Yet, even with such exposure and concomitant enthusiasm, TQM principles have not yet been embraced by most mental health professionals. One of the primary difficulties in translating TQM from manufacturing management to health care management in general, and to behavioral healthcare management in particular, is its lexicon. Psychologists are not used to referring to patients as "customers" or to treatment as a "product," and may initially consider those terms to be in poor taste. Many psychologists consider such a perspective as contrary to the important doctor–patient relationship. However, other TQM terms and models may be a more comfortable fit for psychologists, such as "empowerment," "nonblaming perspectives," "solution-focused goals," "data-based decision making," "working with teams," and "soliciting others' input." and so forth.

Quality and the Business of Practice

Behavioral healthcare practice is indeed a business—be it a facility, group, agency, or solo practice. As people who are in business, leaders, owners, and decision makers must be as cognizant of costs as they are of care. Business, fiscal, and personnel management issues must be equivalent to the clinical aspects of patient care. Although this stance may seem radical, if one cannot stay in business, one cannot provide *any* clinical service. And, if a practice's or facility's support or clinical staff is inappropriate or inefficient, it becomes impossible to provide high-quality care (Stout, in press). The quality of patient care extends well beyond the clinical activities. Billing efficiencies, clerical staff's aid, reception staff's attitudes, and dietary staff's skills are all contributing factors.

Testing Psychologists' Role within TQM

Where do the services of testing psychologists fit within the TQM concepts? It is this author's contention that psychologists are in a strategically key position to help facilities, agencies, or group practices improve their quality of services to their patients and clients. Managed care has actually driven the shift to quality focus by making quality a factor in contracting. (See Chapter 1 for discussion of the evolution of managed care.) In a quality management environment, instead of conducting batteries, testing psychologists will bring their unique psychometric, evaluative, analytic, and reporting skills to bear in assessing quality of service.

Maruish (1991, p. 7) states:

> [P]roblem identification, triage/disposition, and outcome measurement are areas that can greatly affect the success of a mental health organization (be it an agency, hospital, facility, or practice group). There are also areas in which psychological testing can help meet the challenges of the changing healthcare market. Psychometrically based data obtained for the purpose of these functions, along with other data gathered by the organization (e.g., length of treatment for specific disorders, cost of service by unit) can serve as the impetus for action toward quality improvement.

Chapter 2 discussed the use of testing instruments in medical settings, and Chapter 5 detailed outcomes management systems and procedures. Psychometrically rigorous assessment instruments can also be used as:

1. Screening tools.
2. Treatment planning aids.
3. Pre- and posttreatment outcome instruments.

To that list, we now add:

4. Quality management guides.

Outcomes and quality are highly correlated issues in most treatment venues. When outcome results are coordinated with cost data, they become powerful vehicles for managed care contracting purposes, as well as decision-making tools for internal quality improvement. The key is systematic measurement (Maruish, 1991), and testing psychologists hold this key.

To be better positioned to aid in such situations, it is important for psychologists to be aware of the quality procedures, measures, and models that currently exist, and to understand how they work. Volumes have been written on the topic of TQM, and it is beyond the scope of this chapter to provide anything more than an overview. Readers interested in learning more specifics may wish to review publications by Shewart (1939), Howick and Gray (1992), Crosby (1979, 1984), Case (1995), Hinton and Stout (1992), and the National Committee for Quality Assurance (NCQA; 1993). This chapter reviews the relation of TQM to general healthcare (e.g., the "JCAHO Report Card" and the NCQA's HEDIS) and to more specific quality issues that are of concern to behavioral healthcare (e.g., provider profiling and quality indicators).

A Broader Examination of TQM Principles and Methods

Belief systems are key to a systemic adoption of a management style or corporate culture. "Forcing" TQM is antithetical to its own principles and will simply not work. Bergman (1994, p. 46) points out the difference between adopting ideals versus the latest management fad, by asking ". . . employees if they believe in or agree with TQM, and they will (likely) be non-committal. But ask them if they believe that an organization should pay attention to its customers and that employees should understand strategic decisions, and they will quickly agree." The first step in getting behavioral healthcare providers and management to adopt TQM principles is to present the quality control concepts on issues that fit within the existing cultural belief structures. When clinicians get beyond the foreboding language, they will find much that is familiar in the principles of TQM.

Psychologists, in particular, will quickly understand and appreciate the scientific method that TQM principles exploit. For example, decisions are based on collected data, not on hunches, biases, or suppositions; root causes of problems are investigated, with no impulsive intervention based on superficial manifestations; and permanent solutions are sought in lieu of traditional "quick fixes," which are often more problem-causing than problem-solving. These ideas fit the psychological scientist/practitioner's approach quite well. The TQM systems approach, which advocates the examining of the entire organizational gestalt rather than only its independent components, will also be familiar to many clinicians. Only through analysis of the system as a whole can the parts that require attention be identified and improved.

THE 85/15 RULE

A related concept is the 85/15 Rule of "systemic" management (Howick & Gray, 1992, p. 20). By definition, within the 85/15 Rule, 85% of a facility's or practice's problems can be solved by improving the *system*, whereas only 15% of a facility's/practice's problems are within the control of *individuals* within the system. Improvement then results from improving the functioning of the system, instead of blaming the staff.

THE 95/5 RULE

The 95/5 Rule posits that organizational success will result if one deals directly, honestly, and fair-handedly with the 5% of the staff with whom the manager has daily contact. This will have the "pooling" effect of communicating such trust to the remaining 95% of the employees. The point is: staff members function at their optimum when trusted, and the majority of staff come to work (whether at a clinic, facility, agency, practice, or any type of setting) wanting to do a good job, regardless of their duty. Treating others with respect will typically yield respect in return.

PLAN-DO-ACT-CHECK

The concept of Plan-Do-Act-Check aids in operationalizing some of the earlier noted concepts:

- Planning would involve the determination of goals and targets for a current project or task. Developing methods to reach these goals would occur simultaneously.
- Doing would incorporate engaging in any educational or specialized training necessary, then initiating and conducting the work.
- Checking would involve evaluating the effects of implementation and creating a climate for action.
- Acting would involve taking any type of appropriate or necessary action (Crosby, 1979).

COST SAVINGS

Crosby (1979, 1984) notes that the waste that results from poor quality costs an average company approximately 20% of its earnings. Translating this finding to healthcare, the fiscal costs are compounded by the additional risks associated with patients' health status. "Doctors just bury their mistakes" has always been a morbid one-liner, but it makes the point that quality is the sine que non of healthcare.

Couch and Warshaw (1993) extrapolated Crosby's findings to the healthcare industry and projected that approximately $150 million could be saved annually with the application of quality principles and methods. They recommended the following activities as a means to such a quality end (p. 395). Most of these consultative activities are within the practice scope of testing psychologists:

1. Collecting and analyzing data to measure clinician and hospital performance.
2. Modifying internal procedures so that treating patients is, as closely as possible, an error-free process.

142

Among the examples of internal remedial procedures are:

- Instituting stringent quality control programs in all departments and clinics.
- Establishing committees or teams to write research treatment protocols and then monitoring adherence to these protocols.
- Investigating whether consumers and purchasers are satisfied with the programs established to address their concerns.
- Tailoring programs to address health risks and needs of individual insured populations (Couch & Warshaw, 1993).

Testing psychologists' skill with measurement and statistical techniques fits quite closely with these measuring aspects of TQM. The psychologists have expertise in data collection and analysis, measuring performance, making/tailoring procedure recommendations (similar to making treatment recommendations, but on a larger system/scale), measuring satisfaction, and extrapolating/predicting future risk likelihood and its mitigation via preventive measures.

PARETO DIAGRAMMING METHODS

Pareto diagramming is often used to communicate the relationships among factors (Case, 1995). Pareto diagrams can be used with any type of variables; the goals are to investigate, compare, integrate, and reanalyze. The steps in construction are (Case, 1995, p. 68):

1. Identify the problem to be addressed.
2. Select a numerical standard for measurement (e.g., frequencies or cost per day).
3. Select a time period.
4. Graph findings in descending order from left to right on the x-axis.

An example of this method appears in Figure 6.1, which indicates that 70% of the psychological evaluations conducted in the first quarter of calendar year 1995 at ABC Hospital are late (i.e., as defined by

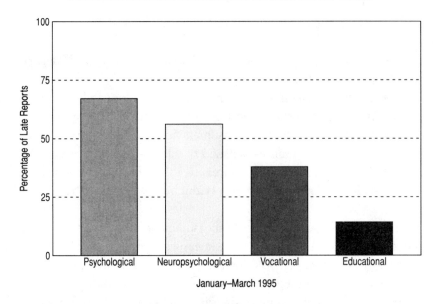

January–March 1995

Timeliness of Evaluations in Patient's Chart
ABC Hospital

FIGURE 6.1
Pareto Diagram

ABC's internally established criterion). In this example, all evaluations are noted along the same scale (percentages), which allows for comparisons.

CAUSE-AND-EFFECT (FISHBONE) DIAGRAMMING

Next, a cause-and-effect or "fishbone" diagram is used to identify the factors associated with testing timeliness (in this example) and its causal relationships with outcomes. An example is depicted in Figure 6.2.

The steps in a fishbone diagram are (Case, 1995, p. 68):

1. List the problem (effect/result).
2. Identify the appropriate major causal areas, and illustrate these as larger "bones."

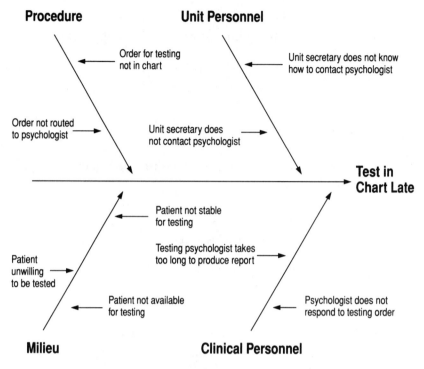

FIGURE 6.2
Fishbone Diagram

3. Deduce the subordinate causes in each major cause through cross-functional teamwork aimed at determining: "Why does this happen?" Note these causes as connected, smaller "bones."

The diagram is used as a method of conceptualizing or crystallizing the problem and its causally related root sources. Each area can be examined discretely, and then as a whole, to identify potential solutions.

After suggested solutions have been articulated and a consensus has been reached, the solutions are "piloted" for a period of time and then reevaluated by the quality team via the same steps (Pareto and fishbone diagrams). If the solutions are working, a longer time interval before the next reevaluation can be established. If they are not working as hoped, new solutions can be developed, piloted, and evaluated. This process continues until satisfactory results are consistently achieved. At that point, further quality enhancements can be considered.

Some Case Examples

Some case examples of TQM in action within the behavioral health arena are provided below.

LATE PROCEDURES IN AN INPATIENT SETTING

Pareto diagramming of evaluation time identified a need for speedier turnaround times of inpatient psychological test reports. The excessive wait for test results was delaying treatment and discharge planning.

A TQM team was developed. Its goal was to decrease the time required to have the results of a complete psychological test battery placed in a patient's chart. First, the Director of Quality Management solicited a team of volunteers who represented all the various "stakeholders" (i.e., people involved in the process) in this area. The team included: the Director of Quality Management (as coach and mentor), a representative unit secretary (the person who routes psychological testing orders), the Director of Staff Development (charged with better orienting staff in the future), a representative of the Medical Records Department (where completed psychological reports are processed, logged in, and then routed to the patients' charts), and a representative testing psychologist who would also function as a TQM consultant. The psychologist was responsible for communicating his or her testing needs (and presumably those of other psychologists as well) and for monitoring and evaluating the new mechanism once it was developed. Ideally, a patient's input might have been used, but it was judged impractical for this task.

The initial meeting included a discussion of the TQM procedure to be utilized, an exploration and common articulation of the problem, and an explanation of how each member normally carried out his or her role or function. A fishbone diagram (see Figure 6.2) served as a graphic. Brainstorming (led by the testing psychologist) was used to develop potential procedures and solutions. A prototype procedure, derived with group consensus, was explicitly written and approved by the group. They then agreed on a six-week pilot test. A meeting was set for the end of the six-week trial, but the team had the option to meet earlier if needed. (An earlier meeting could be called by *any* team member.) The consulting testing psychologist developed a monitoring system to measure the efficacy of the pilot system.

When the six-week trial ended, the team reconvened. The testing psychologist presented results and findings. A few problems were identified, and the group strategized about methods to deal with them. A revised procedure was then tried for another month. At the conclusion of that trial, the team met again, and the psychologist reported on the improved findings. The group members were unanimous in their satisfaction with the revised solution. The new procedure was formally adopted into the hospital's *Quality Management Plan and Policy and Procedure Manual,* and the team was dissolved. The psychologist continued to monitor and report findings on an ongoing basis, allowing for periodic fine-tunings to occur as needed.

PATIENT SATISFACTION

Satisfaction measures are key data in quality improvement initiatives. (Procedures in regard to patient satisfaction were discussed in Chapter 5.) The use of patient satisfaction data for quality measurement and improvement is highlighted in the following example.

TQM principles dictate databased decision making. Patient satisfaction data are critical in determining the quality of a facility's treatment. Thus, an inpatient facility decided to link quality management concerns to patients' opinions. A psychologist with psychometric training developed a patient satisfaction survey from an existing "patient report card." The facility collects patients'

147

responses just prior to discharge and achieves a 70% to 95% patient response rate (a quite favorable rate compared to that of mailed surveys, which typically yield only 2% return rates and provide *poor* generalizability).

The survey data are entered into a database. Each month, the psychologist tabulates the quantitative data and "comment data" (i.e., verbatim patient responses to survey items). The results are compiled and routed to appropriate administrators, directors, and department heads.

Numeric data are generated from Likert Scale items. Annually, using the prior year's aggregate findings, a mean quarterly average and standard deviation are calculated. These averages are used to create an "expected range" of one standard deviation ($\bar{x} \pm 1$ S.D.) above and below the mean. Each quarter's current or "real-time" data are compared with the previous year's benchmark. If a quarter's data fall within the range, the expectation is met. If the data are below the lower range limit of the standard deviation (an indication of patient satisfaction), there is an exploration of what is causally accounting for this improvement (followed by some celebration). If it exceeds the upper range (i.e., showing higher patient dissatisfaction), then it is recommended that a helpful, nonblaming, solution-focused team be formed to help determine the problems and experiment with solutions. The consulting psychologist would act as facilitator of this team. The required statistical procedures are carried out by exporting the database to a statistical packager.

This databased procedure guards against the common retort, "Our department is always in trouble because so-and-so doesn't like us," or its corollary, "That department always gets what it wants because it's *favored*, not because of its performance." For department managers, the systems aid to mitigate anxieties centering around favoritism, antagonism, turf protection, or politics. These are the departments' *own* data—from the patients' perspectives—concerning what is important. Each department is seen as being in the best position to improve its own performance (Hinton & Stout, 1992). In terms of practice expansion, such new, innovative areas are fertile for testing psychologists' expertise.

A Quality Measurement Model for Behavioral Health

TQM lends itself well to all areas of clinical practice. Anderson and Berlant (1994, pp. 139–141) describe a common model in which behavioral health quality issues can be monitored. Consulting testing psychologists can use this model as a theme that allows variations when consulting on TQM issues within a managed care environment. The model has these general areas and concomitant elements:

Utilization Review/Case Management
1. Credentialing/Recredentialing of managers.
2. Clinical rounds participation.
3. Formal supervision by senior clinical staff.
4. Clinical audits of managers' notes, conducted routinely, with feedback.
5. Data tracking (e.g., ALOS by diagnosis) as compared to a benchmark or best-practice standard.
6. Inservice training that is relevant, robust, and ongoing.

Providers
1. Credentialing/Recredentialing following verification of:

    a. License/Certification/Boarding.
    b. Academic history.
    c. Malpractice insurance (at an adequate level).
    d. Malpractice history.
    e. Basic demographic data.
    f. National Practitioner Data Bank affirmation.
    g. Attestations to accuracy of data provided.
    h. Continuing education units.
       (A mechanism that triggers renewal copies of licenses/ malpractice, insurance is recommended.)

2. Case manager ratings of providers as to their:

    a. Cooperativeness.
    b. Quality of care.
    c. Cost effectiveness.

The assessment procedure should be standardized, and clinicians must be aware of the criteria on which they are evaluated.

3. Provider profiling—an examination of cost and utilization of care resources as compared to internal norms or external benchmarks. (More on this later in the chapter.)
4. Treatment change audits—routine evaluations focusing on results and identification of outliers.
5. Provider communications—memos, e-mail, voice mail, updates, newsletters, and other methods to keep practitioners up-to-date with new ideas or procedures that would be helpful.
6. Provider education—remedial and improvement inservices tailored to identified needs.
7. Payor satisfaction surveys—methodological means of sampling managed care organizations' opinions and perspectives.
8. Outcomes monitoring—the issues highlighted in Chapter 5.

A subtle component of such a model would consist of information feedback and cross-checks.

External Evaluations

JCAHO

As noted earlier in the chapter, the Joint Commission on Accreditation of Healthcare Organizations (JCAHO) plays a crucial role in determining and advising on quality issues for the various healthcare organizations it accredits (e.g., mental healthcare programs and facilities, hospitals, nursing homes, healthcare networks, clinical labs, and ambulatory care organizations). Many managed care companies require JCAHO accreditation as a prerequisite for any healthcare organization that seeks to join their network. The evaluative aspect of JCAHO has further expanded into a publicly available Performance Report, colloquially referred to as the "JCAHO Report Card." Interested readers may obtain examples and more detailed information on this process by contacting the JCAHO at One Renaissance Boulevard, Oak Brook Terrace, Illinois 60181; 708-916-5080.

Psychologists with a consultative interest in JCAHO matters should be aware that the reports provide evaluative ratings in the areas of:

1. Assessment of Patients.
2. Behavioral Rehabilitation Services.
3. Chemical Dependency.
4. Diagnostic Radiology Services.
5. Dietary Services.
6. Emergency Services.
7. Governing Body.
8. Improving Organizational Performance.
9. Infection Control.
10. Laboratory.
11. Management and Administration.
12. Management of Information.
13. Medical Staff.
14. Medication Use.
15. Nuclear Medicine.
16. Nursing.
17. Operate Procedures.
18. Organizational Leadership.
19. Patient/Family Rights.
20. Pharmacy.
21. Physical Rehabilitation.
22. Radiation Oncology.
23. Respiratory Care.
24. Safety.
25. Social Services.
26. Special Care.
27. Staff Training.

Psychologists familiar with these areas can have much to offer as consultants.

HEDIS

The National Committee on Quality Assurance (NCQA) has developed a set of measures intended to become a national "benchmark for documenting health plan performance and providing valuable information to both employers and health plans" via the Healthplan Employer Data and Information Set (HEDIS). NCQA continues to develop further refinements and applications of HEDIS. Recently, a "Report Card Pilot Project" was completed, in which measures identified from the HEDIS serve as report card indications for participating health plans.

HEDIS is comprised of five major performance areas, each of which has specific measures. An abbreviated summary of these areas follows (NCQA, 1993, pp. 2–3):

1. Quality.

   Goal: Measure health plans' performance in delivery of certain selected services.

   Preventive Medicine.
   Prenatal Care.
   Acute and Chronic Disease.
   Mental Health—Ambulatory follow-up after hospitalization for major affective disorders.

2. Access and Patient Satisfaction.

   Goal: Measure health plans' performance in providing members access to health care and in satisfying members.

   Access.
   Member Satisfaction.

3. Membership and Utilization.

   Goal: Measure health plans' performance regarding membership stability and demographics, as well as resource allocation with the plan.

   Membership—Enrollment/Dismissal.
   High Occurrence/High Cost.
   Inpatient Utilization (General Hospital/Acute Care).
   Ambulatory Care Utilization.
   Inpatient Utilization (Non-Acute Care).
   Maternity.
   Newborns.
   Mental Health—Treatment on the basis of inpatient, partial, and outpatient location; readmission rate for major affective disorders.

Chemical Dependency—Treatment on the basis of inpatient, partial, and outpatient location; readmission rate for chemical dependency.
Outpatient Drug Utilization.

4. Finance.

   Goal: Measure health plans' performance in achieving financial stability.

   (Fourteen performance measures are specified. They encourage performance, liquidity, efficiency, and compliance with statutory requirements.)

5. Descriptive Information on Health Plan Management and Activities.

   Goal: Assess health plan management and activities.

   (Health plans are encouraged to provide information on many of their other activities—e.g., provider recredentialing, utilization review activities—that can affect members' health, satisfaction, and use of services.)

Although HEDIS currently has a limited focus on behavioral health issues, it will likely expand into this area more fully in the future. Testing psychologists should stay current on industry trends and evaluative issues. In some instances, they may be able to provide consultative assistance in this evaluative domain.

BEHAVIORAL HEALTH REPORT CARDS

AMBHA

The American Managed Behavioral Healthcare Association (AMBHA) is a group comprised of the top managed care organizations in the country. Three working groups report to AMBHA's Quality Improvement and Clinical Services Committees. They are currently developing:

1. A common data set for patient intake.
2. Patient satisfaction methodology.
3. Administrative and clinical indicators leading to the development of a report card (Theis, Geraty, Panzarino, & Bartlett, 1995).

IBH

The Institute for Behavioral Healthcare has developed a National Leadership Council Report Card Task Force charged with comprising a set of behavioral healthcare performance indicators, including minimum data sets and domains (Theis et al., 1995).

CMHS

The Center for Mental Health Services has a Mental Health Statistics Improvement Program that is developing a reporting format focused on: consumer values, primary care, and outcomes. The latter are expanded beyond symptom reduction to include measures of level of functioning and quality of life (Theis et al., 1995).

The report card concept seems to be catching on in all of healthcare. This trend is likely to encourage increased consumer involvement and yield improvements in overall quality. Psychologists can take a contributory as well as a leadership role in this remarkably important and expanding area.

MALCOLM BALDRIGE NATIONAL QUALITY AWARD

Although originally developed for industry, this coveted and prestigious national award is now expanding into healthcare and educational categories. Although healthcare is broadly considered within the categories of the award (Leadership, Information and Analysis, Strategic Planning, Human Resources Development and Management, Process Management, Organizational Performance Results, Satisfaction of Patient and Stakeholders), nothing would prevent a psychiatric hospital or system, a group practice, or an agency from applying for consideration. Qualification is rigorous and demanding, but any behavioral healthcare entity that might win a Baldrige Award would be considered world-class by any standard. Information on Baldrige Award application is available by contacting the National Institute of Standards and Technology at 310-975-2767.

Sources for the leading external evaluation tools are summarized in Table 6.1.

TABLE 6.1
Sources for External Evaluation Tools

American Managed Behavioral
  Healthcare Association
700 13th Street, N.W., Suite 700
Washington, DC 20005
202-434-4565

Evaluative tool: Report Card

Center for Mental Health Services
5600 Fishers Lane, Room 1599
Rockville, MD 20857
301-443-0001

Evaluative tool: Mental Health
  Statistics Improvement Program

Institute for Behavioral Healthcare
4370 Alpine Road, Suite 108
Portola Valley, CA 94028
415-851-6735

Evaluative tool: National Leadership
  Council Report Card

Joint Commission on Accreditation of
  Healthcare Organizations
One Renaissance Boulevard
Oak Brook Terrace, IL 60181
708-916-5080

Evaluative tool: Performance Report

National Committee on Quality
  Assurance
1350 New York Avenue, N.W., Suite
  700
Washington, DC 20005
202-662-1888

Evaluative tool: HEDIS III

National Institute of Standards and
  Technology
Malcolm Baldrige National Quality
  Award
Administrative Building 101, Room
  A537
Gaithersberg, MD 20899-0001
301-975-2767; 301-975-2036

Evaluative tool: Baldrige National
  Quality Award Standards

An Integrated Model

Provider profiling, quality indicators, clinical quality initiatives, and implementation systems considered within a dual context of quality improvement and managed care are current and future concerns for the behavioral healthcare professional, practice, agency, hospital, and system. The following outline integrates the standards of various managed care (Panzarino & Kellar, 1994), association (Kiser, Wagner, & Knight, 1994), practice and facility (Burke, 1992), and accrediting bodies (O'Kane, 1993). This broadband model may include some areas that do not apply to some settings, but it offers a helpful tool for conceptualization. It is provided to aid testing psychologists in becoming more skilled in TQM consultation to various groups. The issues involved in standards for the profession are:

Clinical

1. Credentialing and Recertification Systems for Staff.
2. Performance Indicators:

   - Symptom reduction.
   - Functional improvement.
   - Patient follow-up results.
   - Patient satisfaction.
   - Complaint/Grievance.
   - Patient access to care (provider responsiveness).
   - Adverse occurrence.
   - Documentation quality.
   - Recidivism rates.
   - Efficiency of care provision.
   - Appropriate utilization levels.
   - Compliance to policies and procedures.

3. Standards of Care.
4. Average Length of Stay or Number of Sessions—as cross-tabulated by:

   - Diagnosis.
   - Age, and other patient demographics.

- Provider.
- Site of care.
- Payor.

5. Practice Guidelines.
6. Clinician Satisfaction.
7. Staff Satisfaction.

Fiscal

1. Cost per Case by:

- Provider.
- Diagnosis.
- Treatment site.
- Age group.
- Payor.
- Other relevant demographic data.

2. Cross-Tabulation of Cost-per-Case Data (with the above variables—e.g., cost per case by Dr. Jones for teenage depressed outpatients who have Blue Cross/Blue Shield coverage).
3. Denied/Rejected Claims.
4. New Business Development Efforts.
5. Payor Satisfaction.
6. Cost Efficiency.
7. Cost-Benefit Analysis.
8. Resource Association.
9. Appropriate Utilization.
10. Cost Containment.
11. Payment/Fee Methods and Rates.
12. Viability.
13. Stability.
14. Growth Rate—Actual and Potential.

Operations

1. Admission Criteria.
2. Risk Management and Monitoring Systems.
3. Utilization Management and Monitoring Systems.

4. Quality Management and Monitoring Systems.
5. Adverse Event/Sentinel Monitoring Systems.
6. Management/Administration Capabilities.
7. Community Involvement.
8. Leadership.
9. Mission, Vision, and Values Articulation and Operationalization.
10. Legal Structure.
11. Continuum of Care:

   - Seamless integration of services.
   - Vertical and horizontal integration.

12. Education Initiatives.
13. Client Retention Efforts (when care is needed).
14. Establishment of Benchmarking Standards and Comparative Data:

   - Internal.
   - External.

15. Regulatory and Accreditation Requirements:

   - Council for the Accreditation of Residential Facilities (CARF).
   - Joint Commission on the Accreditation of Health Care Organizations (JCAHO).
   - Health Care Finance Administration (HCFA)
   - Civilian Health and Medical Program of the Uniformed Services (CHAMPUS).
   - State public aid agency.
   - State Department of Public Health.

16. Political/Advocacy Activities.
17. Professional Organization Activities.
18. Stakeholder Input and Systems for Follow-Through.
19. Total Quality Management.

All these areas, although listed discretely, are to be viewed from an integrated perspective; for example, clinical treatment outcomes have an impact on cost data.

Conclusion

Many of the concepts of total quality management and continuous quality improvement involve psychological principles, yet few testing or clinical psychologists apply them to facilities or clinical practices. This situation is likely to change in the future. Managed care's impact in the marketplace has actually played a causal role in driving quality improvement. Testing psychologists are well positioned to offer a great deal to this process because of their unique skills and training in psychometrics, measurement and evaluation, data analysis, reporting mechanisms, and systemic focus.

CHAPTER 7

Risk Management

Many psychologists do not see themselves as being at liability risk. Unfortunately, they are. Risk management deals with identifying legal and ethical pitfalls within psychological practice, and responding to them as necessary. This chapter highlights some of the risks associated with psychological testing and practice, and it reviews the methods to mitigate these risks. The key risk management issue is: A psychologist can be sued even when he or she has not done anything wrong, illegal, or unethical. Cummings and Sobel (1985) noted a case in which a psychologist was sued by the son of a woman he had treated some 20 years before. The son claimed that the psychologist had ruined his childhood because he was unable to successfully treat the mother's depression. The psychologist had never seen or treated the plaintiff.

Need for Tort Reform

Torts are civil lawsuits that are filed in response to alleged harm caused to a plaintiff (e.g., patient) by a defendant (e.g., psychologist). All malpractice suits are torts. The current political focus on tort reform has been born out of some high visibility judgments and growing litigation. Gergen (1991, p. 72) and Quale (1993, p. 24) note:

1. Annually, 18 million new lawsuits enter the U.S. court system.

2. Winning plaintiffs actually receive only about 45% of the amounts awarded. The majority goes to pay attorney fees and court costs.
3. Litigants are tied up for at least 14 months after a suit is filed, and tort cases can stretch on for 5 to 10 years.
4. Lawsuits for malpractice typically involve individuals (e.g., supervisors, unit directors, medical directors, administrators, partners) who may not have had *any* direct contact with the patient-litigant. Yet, every legal charge must be defended, and the emotional and economic costs in such a defense are usually significant.
5. The United States has:

   • Thirty times more lawsuits per person than Japan.
   • Five percent of the world's population, but 70% of its lawyers.

Defense Costs and Specific Malpractice Risks

For mental health practitioners in particular, Heggey (1985) found that, a dozen years ago, the cost of a defense could reach $62,000. More recent statistics (c. 1991, reported by VandeCreek & Stout, 1993) on claims against psychologists note a higher frequency of oc-currences and of associated cases lost. Testing psychologists are at risk for any of the claims listed in Table 7.1. However, they are par-ticularly at risk, because of the testing circumstance, for charges of (VandeCreek & Stout, 1993):

1. Loss from evaluation.
2. Breach of confidentiality.
3. Incorrect diagnosis.
4. Suicide-related claims (e.g., mis- or undiagnosed suicidal intent).
5. Defamation.
6. Loss of child custody and visitation (resulting from a cus-tody evaluation).

TABLE 7.1
Most Frequent Claims against Mental Health Practitioners

Claim	Occurrence	Losses
Sexual misconduct	19%	50%
Incorrect treatment	15	13
Loss from evaluation	11	5
Breach of confidentiality	7	3
Incorrect diagnosis	6	6
Suicide-related claims	6	11
Defamation: libel/slander	4	< 2
Loss of child custody and visitation	3	< 2
Improper meeting of patients	2	< 2

"Triple Crown" of Lawsuits

This author has long noted that psychologists are often at risk for "triple crown" lawsuits: misdiagnosis, failure to treat (because the treatment plan was based on an erroneous diagnosis), and failure to refer (for example, misdiagnosing a thyroid dysfunction as major depression and treating it with cognitive therapy instead of giving a referral to a physician). Because diagnostic testing is often the linchpin to accurate treatment planning, an error in that testing is subsequently amplified and the environment is ripe for liability risk. "Where there's a trauma, there's a tort," has long been a saying in forensic psychology. This author would perhaps add to that: "Where there's a disgruntled client, there's a risk."

Managed Care Risks

DUTY TO APPEAL

Although they are less likely to create a risk for testing psychologists, new case precedents and clinical-legal responsibilities resulting from managed care utilization review procedures are a growing threat.

Numerous legal cases (e.g., *Wickline v. State of California; Warren v. Colonial Penn Franklin Insurance Company; Hughes v. Blue Cross of Northern California; Harrell v. Total Health Care, Inc.; Raglin v. HMO Illinois, Inc.; Boyd v. Albert Einstein Medical Center;* and *Wilson v. Blue Cross of California*) support the contention that the clinician is responsible for determining the course of treatment. Thus, if something goes awry, the clinician will most likely be held culpable. This risk-laden position led to Applebaum's (1993) discussion of psychologists' new "duty to appeal." This concept involves the psychologist in taking steps to appeal any decision or utilization review that the psychologist believes may not be in the best interest of the patient. Applebaum (1993) notes that "clinicians can discharge their fiduciary [in trust] obligations to patients *only* by seeking to persuade others to approve [certain services for] that case" (p. 253). This does not mean that the decision must be overturned before the psychologist's risk can be mitigated. It just means that the psychologist has to exert appropriate effort to try to appeal the decision. Typically, this is not a difficult task. Psychologists have likely appealed utilization reviewers' decisions in the past, and most psychologists feel quite comfortable in the role of patient advocate.

However, some testing psychologists may be surprised to learn that managed care companies can, somewhat arbitrarily, deny payment for services. Some HMOs and other payors argue that they only authorize "payment" for services, not the "provision" (or lack) of services. Testing psychologists are often told: "You can provide any test or compose your testing battery as you wish, but we will only pay for ABC tests or X dollars." The result of this scenario is that ethical psychologists will test as they feel is clinically and ethically warranted by the patient's referral question(s)—despite the distinct possibility that not all of the tests given will be reimbursed.

A caveat is worth noting here. Clinicians may not be alone on this limb much longer. Although not specific to behavioral healthcare, a recent case *(Fox v. Health Network)* established two important legal points (Meszaros, 1994). First, a court ruled *against* a health management organization for denial of services—an important extension of liability to payors. Second, the amount of the award—$89 million including punitive damages—is the largest in such a case in U.S.

legal history. The financial blow was quite sobering to HMOs and the utilization review industry, and may help prevent seemingly random denials of service in the future.

Insurance Fraud Risks

Perhaps one of the most common pitfalls within testing practice is unclear documentation as to who actually conducted the testing procedure, who interpreted the results, and who authored the report. There is no risk of fraudulent billing when all of these procedures are conducted by a licensed and appropriately trained clinical psychologist. Problems become manifest if students, interns, psychometricians, or so-called psychologist-extenders conduct the testing and/or author the report, and their responsibility is not clearly disclosed on the billing statement or report.

Detailed notations of who did what in the testing situation, and the device of having the licensed psychologist sign the report as the supervisor of the author (not as the author) avoid any risk of fraudulent billing or unethical practices. (Supervising a student or technician is fine; the issue of billing inappropriately creates insurance fraud risk.)

Liability Insurance

With the increasing risks posed by managed care practices, adequate liability insurance coverage is a must for all psychologists. Within recent years, many new plans have been developed and offered by insurance carriers, but the plans have created much confusion. The American Psychological Association's Insurance Trust (APAIT, 1994) has developed a guide for clinicians in selecting an insurer and a plan. Copies may be obtained by contacting the APAIT at 800-477-1200.

Contractual obligations (e.g., hold harmless or indemnification clauses) in primary practice organization or managed care organization contracts should always be considered. Errors and omissions coverage and officers' and directors' liability insurance may be necessary for some larger practice groups.

Federal Risks

The good news is that psychological testing can sometimes be federally reimbursed under Medicaid. The bad news is that psychologists must be aware of the anti-kickback laws, safe-harbor violations, and other restrictions under the Stark Amendment. Senator Pete Stark (D, CA) has developed a set of amendments to the federal Medicaid laws that are intended to prevent abuses in the form of inappropriate referral practices. Of primary concern is any "payment for patients." Examples of activities that would be considered violations, as noted by the Office of the Inspector General (OIG, 1993), include:

1. Payment of any type of direct incentive by a hospital each time a psychologist refers a patient to that hospital.
2. Use of free or substantially discounted office space or equipment.
3. Use of free or significantly discounted billing, secretarial, or other staff services.
4. Free training of a psychologist's office staff in areas such as management techniques, Current Procedure Terminology (CPT) coding, billing, and so on.
5. A guarantee that, if a psychologist's income fails to reach a predetermined level, the hospital (or facility) will supplement the remainder up to a certain limit.
6. Low-interest or interest-free loans, or loans that may be "forgiven" if the psychologist refers patients (or some number of patients) to the hospital.
7. Payment of the cost of a psychologist's travel and expenses for attendance at conferences.
8. Payment for a psychologist's continuing education courses.

9. Coverage on a hospital's group health insurance plan, at an inappropriately low cost to the psychologist.
10. Payment for services that require few, if any, substantive duties by the psychologist, or payment for services in excess of their fair market value.

These restrictive rules are intended to prevent hospitals (or other state or federally funded facilities) from offering any type of incentive that could influence a provider to "steer" a patient to a facility for a fiscal reason not a clinical necessity. Violators are subject to criminal prosecution under the Medicare and Medicaid anti-kickback statutes.

Patient Risk Factors

Kull (1989) has identified ten warning signs that may indicate liability risks:

1. A disgruntled patient.
2. A dissatisfied family.
3. A deteriorating patient/clinician relationship.
4. Adverse reports from a patient representative (for inpatient cases).
5. An embittered guarantor.
6. A routine outpatient review in which comprehensiveness and appropriateness of diagnosis and treatment are unexpectedly challenged.
7. Pharmacy concerns.
8. Incomplete medical records.
9. Patients who fall outside of facility procedures for passes, privileges, elopement, and other activities.
10. Incident reports.

Not all of these warning signs may directly impact testing psychologists, but because most malpractice suits name multiple defendants, psychologists (particularly those working on multidisciplinary treatment teams) must be vigilant about indirect risks.

Documentation Issues

Because a psychologist can never be certain that a report, data, or file may not be used against him or her in litigation, it is important to keep the following recommendations in mind:

1. Never, under any circumstances, alter a patient's record or report. Addenda are certainly appropriate if done in a legitimate and timely fashion. Not only is it illegal and unethical to alter patient records, it is usually futile to try. Since the 1980s, the Internal Revenue Service (IRS) has required that inks manufactured in the United States must be formulated with trace chemicals that vary from year to year. A simple forensic chemical analysis of a written document can pin down, with considerable certainty, when it was written (and whether it was later altered). Electronic or computer-based files are also easily evaluated for authenticity or alteration.
2. Some things are not appropriate to include in a report, file, or clinical note. Taboo topics (Bales, 1987; Kull, 1989; Negley, 1985; Soisson, VandeCreek, & Knapp, 1987) include:

   - Hunches.
   - Value judgments.
   - Emotional statements (on the psychologist's part, e.g., "The patient's tenor was quite trying/upsetting/angering/etc. today . . .").
   - Personal opinions that are irrelevant to diagnosis or treatment.
   - Illegal behavior (on the client's part) that is not homicidal or suicidal.
   - Sexual practices that are irrelevant to the clinical picture.

- So-called "sensitive information," which holds little clinical utility and which could, if made public (via court order or proceeding), embarrass or cause harm to the patient or others.

Record Keeping

Some managed care circumstances raise additional ethical considerations of breaching confidentiality. It is always incumbent for the testing clinician to review any type of contractual language or consent forms regarding the release of psychological test data, psychological testing reports, or computer-generated reports, to a managed care company or to a utilization reviewer.

The American Psychological Association (APA) recommends that clinicians keep their records of a testing case, including any raw data or notes for at least three years. A summary of the record should be kept for twelve years.

This author recommends keeping the entire test record, including raw data, in perpetuity. The reason is that the statute of limitations does not actually "start ticking" until it is clear to the patient that harm has been done. In an extreme example, twenty years could pass and a clinician could then be involved in a suit. Having archived records could mean the difference between being prepared and being in trouble. The volume of materials versus available storage space and costs may require some special arrangements for off-premises archiving.

Exemptions to Confidentiality

The whole point of patient confidentiality is to ensure the patient's right to privacy. Most states articulate very clearly the parameters for confidentiality, but there are some exceptions, specifically:

1. *Workers' compensation law.* This law supersedes mental health law in most states. The reason is best explained via an example. If a workers' compensation claim is lodged against an employer for something that has involved psychological testing, the employer's not having access to the report would be tantamount to a denial of the employer's constitutional right to prepare a defense (i.e., due process).

2. *Patient request.* If a patient requests a copy of any type of test report, that report can be released to him or her. This does not include raw test data, or any type of personal notes per se. It continues to be unethical to release any type of raw test data to anyone who is not properly trained to be able to interpret those data. Some individuals consider computer-generated reports analogous to raw data rather than completed psychological reports. From this perspective, there would be a reason for not releasing psychological tests that are computer-scored, and the resultant reports. Most reports that are generated by computers indicate that they should not be released because of the problematic nature of such tests and findings. The best clinical policy is to not release a copy of a computer test report to the patient or to untrained clinical individuals.

3. *Consent of the patient.* This varies from a request by virtue of the fact that a patient can consent for a psychological report, or any part of a clinical record, to be sent to anyone else. It may not be in the patient's best interest, and the psychologist can make that known to the patient. Nevertheless, the patient has the final say regarding any reports that are sent out with that patient's consent.

4. *Laws requiring disclosure.* In certain circumstances, state law mandates breach of confidentiality. For example, child abuse or elder abuse must be reported. In the State of Illinois, it is a Class A Misdemeanor if a clinician has not reported a suspicion, an evidence, or an allegation of any type of child abuse to the appropriate authorities within twenty-four hours of learning of it.

5. *Medicare and Medicaid laws.* These laws supersede confidentiality acts for reporting of information.

6. *If the patient is a litigant.* If a lawsuit is filed against a psychologist, the patient cannot claim that confidentiality has been breached when the clinician must disclose information relevant to his or her defense of the suit.

7. *Duty-to-warn or duty-to-protect laws.* Although not every state recognizes the Tarasoff Doctrine established in California, most states have a duty-to-warn law: A clinician must inform the target if a patient reports a homicidal ideation. Similarly, duty-to-protect laws require informing appropriate individuals that an identified patient is perhaps homicidal, or suicidal, and that measures may need to be taken for involuntary hospitalization.

8. *Future criminal behavior.* This is a remarkably vague area and a legal "minefield" for clinicians. A clinician is best advised to rely on duty-to-warn and duty-to-protect concepts, or the Tarasoff Doctrine, with regard to future criminal behavior that may create risk of harm to other individuals or self-harm to the patient. (This situation may manifest among individuals who deal in the sale and distribution of drugs and are being tested, or are in treatment, for drug or substance abuse.) In instances where the intent is not clear, the best recommendation is to seek clinical supervision and consultation on the case, in addition to legal advice.

9. *Any type of emergency.* If an individual is in need of immediate medical care, or if there is a medical emergency or a need for commitment procedures, the situation takes precedence over confidentiality concerns.

10. *Within the context of supervision.* Most laws allow individuals in a supervisor–supervisee relationship to share confidential patient information.

11. *A court order.* This intervention varies from state to state. Some states require breaching of confidentiality at the subpoena level. However, other states do *not* allow release of information in response to a subpoena, unless it is accompanied by a signed patient consent. The only circumstance in which

a record can be released, in some states, is when a court order is obtained. In effect, it is a subpoena signed by a judge. Figure 7.1 is a sample response to a subpoena in states that require a court order for release of confidential information.

12. *Federal grand jury subpoena.* If a patient is the focus of an investigation and a clinician's records are judged to have possible bearing in the matter, then this type of subpoena may be issued. The clinician must release what is requested.

13. *IRS subpoena.* As with a federal grand jury subpoena, if a client may be suspected by the IRS of conducting illegal activities in tax matters, and if, for some reason, the clinician may have information relevant to an investigation, records must be released.

Practice Recommendations

"Pleased patients seldom sue." A bit of empathy and responsivity can go a long way toward the goal of having some pleased patients. Psychologists should communicate that their patients' opinions and perspective are valued. Some additional practice recommendations include (Bales, 1987; Kull, 1989; Negley, 1985; Soisson et al., 1987):

1. Secure informed consent from the patient if competent, or from a guardian if the patient is adjudicated incompetent.

2. Clarify the clinical procedures and activities. Note risks/rewards and incorporate the active participation of the patient where clinically appropriate.

3. Be clear as to personal limits and expertise. Refer when indicated. Do not practice outside of professional scope.

4. Consult with colleagues on difficult cases, and episodically. Enter the consultation in the clinical record but maintain patient confidentiality and anonymity.

5. Stay up-to-date with current practices and diagnostic techniques. Incompetence is a poor defense.

IN THE CIRCUIT COURT OF YOUR COUNTY, ILLINOIS

IN THE INTEREST OF)
)
)   GENERAL NUMBER:
)
alleged to be   )
A MINOR   )

RESPONSE TO SUBPOENA

TO: Sally S. Smith   Robert M. Billing
     Clerk of the Circuit Court Attorney for Your Patient
     Your County, Illinois
     Hard Knox Juvenile Complex
     1000 Grand Avenue
     City, State 60000

I decline to testify or produce the records and documents described in, and in response to, the subpoena received by me by Certified Mail on January 29, 1997, in the above matter, returnable to the Honorable Judge Jones or Judge Presiding at Hard Knox Juvenile Complex, 1000 Grand Avenue, City, State, on five days after service, by virtue of the provisions and prohibitions of Sections 3, 4, 5, and 10 of the Mental Health and Disabilities Confidentiality Act, any other applicable sections thereof, and any other applicable laws.

Dated: February 2, 1997   ASSOCIATES

                                           BY: _____
                                                Owner

I served this Response to Subpoena by mailing a signed copy to Sally S. Smith, Clerk of the Circuit Court of Your County, Illinois, and Robert M. Billing, at the above address, via Certified Mail P 123 456 789 and P 987 654 321, respectively, postage prepaid, on April 1, 1997.

                                           _____
                                           Office Manager

Signed and Sworn before me
on April 1, 1997

_____
Notary Public

FIGURE 7.1
Sample Response to a Subpoena
Source: Judith Claxton, Claxton & Associates, Crystal Lake, IL.

6. Utilize patient satisfaction measures to gain ideas and feedback as to what might be initiated to improve patients' satisfaction levels. (See Chapters 5 and 6 for more on patient satisfaction.)
7. Keep complete, accurate, appropriate notes that are never altered.
8. Follow up when any unusual or atypical incidents occur, and document having done so.
9. Be vigilant regarding personal communication, style, and attitude toward the patient. Be equally vigilant about the patient's communication, style, and attitude in return.
10. Be cautious of any patient who evidences a great like or dislike in his or her responses or reactions.
11. Never include personal revelations in conversations with a patient.
12. Rarely (if ever) touch a patient.
13. Do not try to collect on past-due bills with borderline patients.
14. Obtain the patient's written consent to talk to any past therapists or to obtain past reports or clinical notes.
15. Document all diagnostic decisions and rule-out rationales.
16. Use extreme caution in the evaluation (or treatment) of patients diagnosed with repressed traumatic memories, post-traumatic stress disorder (PTSD), Borderline Personality Disorder (BPD), Multiple Personality Disorder (MPD), paranoia or paranoid dependent personality disorder, personality disorders, or sexual problems.
17. Take notes and write reports as if they will someday be read as evidence for the prosecution.
18. Retain records forever.

Issues with regard to malpractice obviously do not solely lie in the domain of treatment. Pope and Vasquez (1991) notes "Figures compiled by the *APA Insurance Trust* comprising all malpractice suits closed over a twelve-year period indicate that incompetent or improper assessment techniques are the fifth most frequent cause of suits against psychologists, accounting for about 3.7 percent of the total costs and about 5.4 percent of the total number of claims" (p. 2). Pope offers these recommendations to help mitigate testing psychologists' risk:

1. Keep current; failure to do so can lead to malpractice.
2. Clients' reading level must be adequate for the instrument.
3. Norms commonly used with a test may not fit a particular assessment task or client.
4. Test administration must be adequately monitored.
5. Standardized tests are for use in a standardized manner.
6. Factors that may affect the meaning of test findings must be formally reported.
7. Test results are hypotheses.

If a Suit Is Filed

As noted earlier, there is not always a correlation between wrongdoing and lawsuits. Thus, some psychologists who have done nothing wrong may find themselves in the awkward, upsetting posture of a defendant. *Psychotherapy Finances* (1994, pp. 7–8) provided these steps, to be undertaken if needed:

1. Recognize this is an all-too-common occurrence. You just have been snagged.
2. Don't panic, but don't underreact either.
3. Contact your attorney.
4. Contact your liability insurance carrier.
5. Follow their instructions without a fault.
6. Do not talk about it to others. Period. Although this may seem antithetical to psychologists to not "share," lawsuits become public quickly enough, and loose talk can damage a reputation. Moreover, friends one speaks with could be brought into court as plaintiff's witnesses if given details relevant to the case. Keep in mind: From the time you are served until

the case is resolved or adjudicated, anything you say can and will be brought into the courtroom by the plaintiff's attorney.

7. Collect all records that relate to the case, including files, calendars, clinical notes, reports, raw data, billing records, and so forth.
8. Never alter anything.
9. Develop a witness list for the *attorney* to follow up with—*not* you.
10. Do not go to the plaintiff and attempt to "work things out." This will usually backfire and make things worse.
11. Be prepared for the "long haul" to get to the case's end.

Response Model to an Investigation

Simply by virtue of being in practice, all psychologists face the risk of litigation. Although the steps outlined in this chapter will help mitigate the risk of lawsuits, nothing can fully ensure against a claim being filed. Thus, it is equally important to know what to do if an investigation is initiated. Crick (1990) has outlined the following annotated steps (pp. 4–5, reprinted with permission):

1. *Do not provide any information via telephone.* Even with caller ID technology, it is not possible to know exactly who is on the other end of the line. It is best to keep all communications via correspondence or in person to any opposing party.
2. *Verify the identity of the investigator and the agency.* Ask for some type of identification, be it a business card, badge, identification card, or driver's license. Find out the position of the person or title (e.g., server, investigator, attorney, state employee, etc.).
3. *Determine if **you** are the focus of the investigation.* You may be involved as a witness, not the ultimate defendant. (If you are the focus, seek legal counsel's assistance prior to responding to any questions.) If you are not the focus of investigation, request a letter (or some document) attesting to that effect.
4. *Request to have someone else present in the interview.*

5. *Try to learn what exactly the inquiry or investigation is about.* If at any time you feel that you are at risk in any manner, stop the interview at that point and obtain a legal consult from your attorney.

6. *Never lie.* If you are unsure or do not know the answer to a question, do not answer with an assumption. If you are unsure, just say so. You may feel that every question should be answerable, but not all are. Do not feel pushed into a corner or that a little lie will not come back to haunt you.

7. *If you are told at any time in the investigation that "you have the right to remain silent,"* do so, and immediately obtain legal counsel. You have just been Mirandized and are subject to criminal investigation procedures. It would be best to then not say anything more until your counsel arrives. You may ask if you are free to go or if you are under arrest.

8. *If you are the focus of investigation, unless instructed otherwise by counsel:*
   • Do not provide original or copies of any documents, files, notes, etc., unless you have been served with a court corder or a search warrant.
   • Do not identify, acknowledge, or provide comment or opinion on any documents shown to you.
   • Do not provide or sign any written statements.

9. *If any documents, computers or disks, or any other materials* are seized by a court order or search warrant, obtain a detailed receipt for them.

10. *Be wary of any so-called "informal" or "informational" conferences you are asked to attend.* Specifically ask the nature, structure, intent of the meeting, and who else is to be attending.

General Recommendations

Accusations of malpractice or unethical conduct can create high levels of panic and fear. These emotional responses may be misjudged as signs of guilt by the opposing party. It is therefore important to work through attorneys. Advocacy is what they are trained to do. Law is quite different from psychology or science in its fundamental approach to arriving at truth. In science, truth is presumed to be discovered via replicability and probability (e.g., 95% certainty or p = .05). In law, the truth of fifty years may change tomorrow via a new case precedent. The adversarial process of law is also typically alien and antithetical to the collaborative, compromising, consensus-seeking style of psychologists. Although it's natural to solicit emotional support through such a trying ordeal, it is also important to keep in mind the possibility that any discussions or conversations may be introduced as testimony in court. As unfair as this may seem, it is quite possible. Never underreact to any legal threat. Immediately assume a fact-finding defensive posture. Frivolous cases are more rapidly quashed with immediate, strong, defensive responses.

It will also bode well, in both quality clinical practice and in any legal circumstance, to maintain some type of documented supervisory or peer review process in which a participant gains additional ideas or suggestions from peers or a mentor. If involved in such a group or relationship, others can lend perspective, providing early warning signs for high-risk cases. If a case becomes legally problematic, documentation of other professionals' input on the circumstances (not the identities) in the case can be tremendous support for the clinical/diagnostic decisions made.

For the testing psychologist, it is especially important to be able to justify (if ever necessary) all diagnostic decisions made. This implies adequate training in general (psychometrics, psychopathology, and psychodiagnostics) and specific knowledge of the types of cases seen (e.g., child, substance abuse, medical, forensic, and so on). It is important to be thoroughly conversant with the DSM and to be able to articulate a differential psychodiagnostic process along with a theoretical orientation (with its inherent strengths and weaknesses).

It is crucial to maintain appropriate limits, boundaries, and roles. Although most psychologists are friendly, warm, and empathic, it is incumbent for clinicians to make sure that those attributes are not misperceived as anything more. There should be no social, business, or any other extraclinical contacts with patients. This temptation is sometimes exacerbated by the testing circumstance; some erring psychologists think that if the clinical relationship is circumscribed to "only testing," there is no harm in other nonclinical contact or activities. This is simply not the case. The clinical relationship established by testing consultation is no different than that of psychotherapy. All rules, responsibilities, and boundaries are the same.

Testing consultations are often expensive, and, within managed care, they are frequently not fully (if at all) paid for. Billing patients who do not intend to pay for the consultation, or sending a case to collections often triggers the patient to file a frivolous suit as a countermeasure. The patient's manipulative strategy is that the suit will be dropped if the bill is also dropped. Akin to blackmail, the tactic reminds one of the cliché, "The best defense (against paying a bill) is a good offense (file an unfounded suit)." Psychologists should be wary of this possibility in the decision-making process involving how and whom to bill. Often, when collection agencies are used, the suit filed will charge a breach of confidentiality. A preventive mechanism is to have an office policy requiring all patients to sign a document in which they acknowledge knowing that unpaid bills may go to collectors.

Conclusion

As this chapter noted initially, tort reform is occurring, but it is not a panacea. It remains the testing psychologist's responsibility to practice within strict parameters, and to not hesitate in seeking legal counsel where needed. Applying the principles in this chapter—and staying current with ethical, legal, regulatory, and assessment/ diagnostic standards—may not prevent a lawsuit, but it should help foster a solid defense.

CHAPTER 8

Medical Cost Offset

T HIS CHAPTER FOCUSES ON the medical cost reductions that can be realized with early psychological interventions. Medical cost offset refers to the savings from an individual's avoidance of medical care as a result of receiving timely psychological care. For example, it is far less expensive to successfully treat alcohol addiction (e.g., $20,000) than to replace an addict's liver ($200,000). The amount saved is the "offset" ($180,000). Four sources of such offsets are generally considered to be afforded by psychology:

1. Psychological problems that become manifest in primary care (e.g., depression).
2. Certain medical problems that have a robust psychological basis (e.g., hypertension, gastrointestinal problems, liver disease).
3. Dually diagnosed/concomitant medical and psychological disorders (e.g., heart attack and depression).
4. Treatment compliance in general medical patient populations (e.g., smoking cessation, sobriety, weight loss).

The concepts, studies, and findings presented here provide material that can be used in the development of programs or marketing plans. Readers can then tailor specific programs for various medical practice or facility settings. The information provided is intended to assist in both structuring programs and marketing them, in order to yield maximum benefit in patient care while acting responsibly toward the fiscal issues that accompany any medical treatment decisions.

Who Needs Behavioral Health?

CARVE-OUTS AND HIDDEN DOLLAR COSTS

Initially, managed care's focus on cost reduction gave rise to the "carve-out" phenomenon—the removal of the behavioral health benefit from a general medical benefit package. MCOs were responding to a common employer position: "None of my employees is crazy, so why do I need this extra cost?" Knowing that employees expect a general medical benefits package, a vision plan, and a dental plan, many employers felt that behavioral health packages only added unnecessary costs. More sophisticated employers understand that decreasing behavioral health benefits leads to an *increase* in other healthcare costs. For example, the hidden costs of behavioral illness include:

1. Poor decision making on an employee's part.
2. Damage to a company's public image (when someone does something that gains negative notoriety in the media or within the company itself).
3. High personnel turnover (including the costs of recruiting and training new staff) as well as diverted supervisory and managerial time.
4. Friction among workers, which negatively impacts productivity.
5. Risk of damage to equipment.
6. Risk of damage to other staff members' morale.

REAL DOLLAR COSTS

These issues convert into real dollar costs. A company's unmet behavioral health treatment needs can result in:

1. Increased absenteeism.
2. Increased tardiness.
3. Increased sick leave.
4. Increased overtime pay for those who have to carry the absentees' burden of the workload.
5. Increased on-site injuries and accidents.
6. Increased workers' compensation claims.
7. Increased costs for security.
8. Increased premiums for subsequent medical insurance.

ECONOMIC IMPACT

Looking at the issue of medical cost offset on a larger scale, the economic loss associated with mental and addictive disorders is dramatic. Price and Cisco (1985) placed the annual total loss at $273.3 billion a decade ago. Of this total, 36% ($98.4 billion) was spent on treatment-related costs, and 24% ($65.6 billion) went toward closing the gap that resulted from reduced employee productivity. Another 24% of lost earnings was attributable to premature deaths, and 16% ($43.7 billion) resulted from law enforcement, fire departments, and similar costs. Approximately $37 million are lost annually as a result of poor productivity. Other work issues have equally starting statistics:

- Industrial accidents—80% to 90% are related to personal problems, not to competency nor inherent risks associated with the employee's position.
- Absences—61% result from psychological problems.
- Termination of employment—65% to 80% of dismissals occur because of employees' personal problems, not poor job performance nor incompetence.

BEHAVIOR DISORDER PREVALENCE

Psychiatric and substance abuse disorders are serious and prevalent. Jansen (1986) noted that almost 48 million adults have experienced at least one diagnosable psychiatric disorder in their lifetime. In any given year, mental disorders affect an average of 40.7 million American adults or 22% of the American population, according to statistics provided by the National Institute of Mental Health (NIMH) and the National Advisory Mental Health Council (NAMHC). Almost one-third of these individuals have symptoms for a full year or longer, and more than one-third report some disability associated with the mental disorder. Severe mental disorders (for example, schizophrenia, manic depression, bipolar disorder, suicidal levels of depression, panic disorder, and obsessive-compulsive disorder) affect 5 million people (or 2.8% of the American adult population). Substance abuse disorders affect 17.5 million Americans (or 9.5% of the adult population) in any given year.

According to Regier, Narrow, and Rae (1993), one-third of Americans have suffered from mental and addictive disorders without receiving any treatment. Yet, some employers and payors believe that behavioral healthcare issues are inconsequential, and that treatment for such disorders typically is "expensive hand-holding." Psychotherapy was frequently misunderstood as being a purchased friendship as opposed to serious treatment on a par with medical specialties. The diagnostic aspects of the presence of a psychiatric disorder were viewed by some as resulting from an inherent weakness in the individual rather than a true "disorder."

BEHAVIOR HEALTH/MEDICAL CROSS-OVER AND WASTE

According to research compiled by the Georgia Psychological Association, HMO studies confirm the overuse of primary care physicians for behavioral health problems. Of the patients occupying general hospital beds, 25% to 40% are actually being treated for complications of alcoholism. Alcoholic individuals' use of health services is four times that of nonalcoholics. These issues open into a broader picture when the families of alcoholics are included. These family members incur twice as many medical costs as families of nonalcoholic individuals. Seventy-three percent of patients admitted to general hospitals for head trauma have alcohol in their bloodstream, and 58% of traumatic brain injury survivors have a history of substance abuse. Persons who have no identifiable physical illness use 30% to

60% of all physician visits; these people develop physical symptoms because of unmanaged emotional stress. Primary care physicians and HMO gatekeeper physicians have an obvious overutilization of their time and services for dealing with behavioral health issues. With early intervention as a result of early assessment via psychological screening, these costs can be controlled and reduced.

EMPLOYER AND SOCIETAL WORRY

On a broader scale, employers have additional worries, such as the fact that 70% of all illegal drug users are currently employed, and 1 out of 12 full-time employees reports current illicit drug use.

A recent page-one article in the *Wall Street Journal* (January 3, 1995) noted that, from 1989 to 1992, First Chicago Bank employees took an average of 40 days off per employee because of depression. This is a higher rate of absenteeism than for "back pain, heart disease, high blood pressure, diabetes, and other mental health ailments." Half of First Chicago's mental health claims are for depression treatment—in comparison, for example, to 7% for alcohol and drug abuse. Many large firms are starting to recognize and respond to this problem. General Motors, Texaco, and other companies are providing their employee assistance programs with funding for a "depression kit"—an aid to uncovering depression.

Society also needs to worry. Untreated substance abuse accounts for 65% of spousal beatings, 55% of physical child abuse reports, 65% of murders, and 88% of knifings.

Behavioral Healthcare's Impact

For individuals who complete successful substance abuse treatment, medical healthcare costs quickly decline to a level that is normal for nonalcoholic individuals. A concomitant reduction occurs in the physical healthcare needs and costs of the treated alcoholic's spouse and family, even though they may never have been involved in the treatment or identified as patients (Georgia Psychological Association, 1991).

EMPLOYER SAVINGS

Workplace savings can accrue from increases in productivity, decreases in absenteeism and accidents, reduced attrition and turnover, and the associated costs. Marked cost reductions can result if employees who are in need of care are referred to behavioral health specialists early—prior to greater symptomatic presentation of their problems.

TESTING'S ROLE

Certain screening instruments (noted in Chapters 2 and 3) and methods for instituting screening procedures can help employers monitor behavioral healthcare problems resulting from unmanaged stress, work-related issues, or substance abuse problems. Early identification is helpful in finding current employees who are candidates for early intervention or Employee Assistance Program (EAP) services—perhaps prior to problems of absenteeism, injuries, and workers' compensation claims. (Such screening can be considered for hiring decisions, as long as it does not violate state laws and the Americans with Disabilities Act.)

An inaccurate diagnosis, or an undiagnosed additional disorder, can have a chain reaction. A patient's length of stay in a facility, or the number of sessions for an outpatient, will increase, and one additional week of inpatient care could cost thousands of dollars. Unnecessarily long treatment is not quality patient care. Misuse of medical care while attempting to treat an undiagnosed psychological disorder increases both treatment costs and liability risks.

Treatment Efficacy

Psychological treatment works. The efficacy of many treatments for severe mental disorders is comparable to that of other branches of medicine, including surgery. According to the National Advisory Mental Health Council (Goodwin & Moskowitz, 1993), over a six-month period, two heart procedures, angioplasty and atherectomy, had treatment success rates of 41% and 52%, respectively. Both are well below the early-response success rates of treatments for some of the most severe mental illnesses. For example, schizophrenia holds a 50% treatment-management success rate, and obsessive-compulsive disorder has a treatment success rate of 60%. Appropriate treatment planning and beneficial treatment outcome are the results of appropriate assessment, diagnosis, and triage. The impact of appropriate treatment is manifold and marked.

BIPOLAR DISORDER

Without care, individuals with bipolar disorder typically spend one-fourth of their adult lives in hospitals and fully one-half of their lives disabled (National Association of Psychiatric Healthcare Systems [NAPHS], 1994). These statistics are important for managed care companies. Effective medications (lithium carbonate, and anticonvulsants for lithium-resistant patients) are often used in combination with supportive, directive psychotherapy. This produces a 75% to 80% efficacy rate for the treatment of bipolar-disordered individuals who can then lead essentially normal and productive lives.

MAJOR DEPRESSIVE DISORDER

Antidepressant medications have been effective in approximately two-thirds of individuals with major depressive disorders (NAPHS, 1994). Success rate of treatment increases to 85% when alternative or adjunctive medications are used alone or in combination with psychotherapy. Psychotherapy alone helps some depressed individuals, especially those with mild to moderate symptomatology. Major depression accounts for more "bed days" (people out of work and in bed) than any other "physical disorder" with the exception of cardiovascular disorders. Major depression is more costly to the economy than chronic respiratory illness, diabetes, arthritis, or hypertension. Major depression is among the most common clinical problems encountered by primary care physicians, and is often one of the most underdiagnosed or misdiagnosed. (Refer to Chapter 3 for a full discussion of accurate diagnosis of depression and a methodology to aid in the differential diagnosis of a physical disorder mimicking depression. Chapter 2 gives other screening tools.)

PANIC DISORDER

Effective treatment options (including traditional antidepressants and high-potency antianxiety agents) and refinements of behavioral psychotherapies have brought the effective treatment response rates to 70% to 90% of individuals diagnosed with panic disorder (NAPHS, 1994). Somatic symptoms of panic disorder often confound the diagnostic process and lead to unnecessary expenditure of healthcare resources (e.g., unnecessary angiograms performed because of panic-disorder symptoms: racing heartbeat, difficulty in breathing, chest pains, and dizziness mimicking cardiac distress). Costs associated with misdiagnosis are more than $32 million annually.

POSTSURGICAL CONSULTATION

Psychotherapy provided postoperatively for various surgical procedures has consistently decreased the length of general hospital inpatient stays and has demonstrated concomitant improvement of patient prognosis (Mumford et al., 1984; Wiggins, 1994). Behavioral healthcare rehabilitation has been estimated to produce a cost benefit ratio in excess of 12:1. For every $1.00 spent for behavioral healthcare rehabilitation, a savings of $12.00 in subsequent healthcare costs has resulted. Testing psychologists' roles would gain best advantage in differential diagnostic procedures.

Psychology's Interface with Mortality Rates

Of the fifteen leading causes of death (National Cancer Center for Health Statistics, 1993), heart disease, the number-one cause, can

benefit from psychological care administered for prevention and rehabilitation (Wiggins, 1994). The same benefit is associated with cancer
and stroke. Chronic obstructive pulmonary disease can be mitigated
by psychological care in the realm of prevention, intervention, and rehabilitation. When applied to rehabilitation issues, psychological care
can positively impact accidents, pneumonia and flu, and diabetes. Prevention, intervention, and rehabilitation are helpful in decreasing
successful suicides, the eighth leading cause of death. Prevention and
rehabilitation can also impact the spread of HIV infection. Prevention, intervention, and rehabilitation have demonstrated positive
impacts on decreasing homicide rates, liver disease, and cirrhosis. Additionally, nephritis, nephrotic syndrome, and nephrosis can be han-
dled with psychological rehabilitation. And, perinatal problems can be
reduced by psychological care via prevention and rehabilitation (Wiggins, 1994).

Psychology's Role in the Most Frequently Diagnosed Medical Problems

An examination of healthcare costs, early assessment, and triage issues of the 20 principal diagnoses of patients of all ages, as identified
by frequency of visits to primary care physicians, indicates that 16
diagnoses, or 80%, are behaviorally related (Wiggins, 1994) (see
Table 8.1).

Accurate Patient Identification

For any medical cost offset to be realized, patients must first be appropriately identified. This is the function of testing psychologists.
Prior to psychologists' evaluation, however, medically trained professionals (e.g., primary care physicians, internists, family practitioners,
general practitioners) may be the first persons to whom these patients present. (Screening tools for these medical professionals are

TABLE 8.1
Principal Diagnoses of Patients of All Ages, Ordered by Frequency of Visits to Primary Care Physicians

Rank	Diagnosis
1.	Essential hypertension.*
2.	Acute upper respiratory infection of multiple or unspecified types.
3.	General medical examination.*
4.	Suppurative and unspecified otitis media.
5.	Diabetes mellitus.*
6.	Acute pharyngitis.*
7.	Chronic sinusitis.*
8.	Bronchitis, not specified as acute or chronic.
9.	Normal pregnancy.
10.	Sprains/Strains of other and unspecified parts.*
11.	Other and unspecified disorders of the back.*
12.	Allergic rhinitis.
13.	Health supervision of infant or child.*
14.	Other disorders of the urethra and urinary tract.*
15.	General symptoms.*
16.	Obesity and other hyperalimentation.*
17.	Asthma.*
18.	Osteoarthosis and allied disorders.*
19.	Contact dermatitis and other eczema.*
20.	Acute tonsillitis.

* Behaviorally related diseases.
Source: G. Schmitting (Ed.). (1993). *Facts about Family Practice* (p. 66). Kansas City, MO: American Academy of Family Physicians. Copyright 1993 by American Academy of Family Physicians. As cited in Wiggins, (1994).

discussed in detail in Chapter 2.) Testing psychologists will likely need to alter their testing batteries to deal with populations having:

1. Medical problems without concomitant psychopathology.
2. Medical problems with co-morbidity of psychopathology.
3. No actual medical problem, but psychopathological problems.

Testing psychologists may always select instruments within a particular battery, based on the referral data or discernible patient factors (e.g., demographics). Chapter 3 examines specialized medical populations and more fully discusses test selection and procedures as well as methodologies for differential diagnostic evaluations between biological and psychological etiologies.

GENERAL SCREENING TOOL

Kessler, Cleary, and Burke (1985) utilized the General Health Questionnaire (an interview-based tool) with 1,072 medical patients in a primary care clinic. The questionnaire was used as a screening method for identifying which patients had a diagnosable mental disorder. The procedure is an efficient, nondisruptive practice enhancement and could easily serve as an initial component of a more fully executed battery, if indicated, or simply as a helpful screening device. (The researchers found that 35% of the patients screened with the General Health Questionnaire had some type of psychopathology.)

The General Health Questionnaire was also used by Brody (1980) in an inpatient medical/surgical hospital setting with 235 patients undergoing long-term medical intervention. The profiles held by the questionnaire indicated that 63% (N = 149) had findings suggestive of the presence of a psychological disorder. Thus, it is important for testing psychologists to be sensitive to and aware of which tests are appropriate for the various treatment venues. Instruments that can be flexibly and reliably used in most medical case contexts should be selected.

Marketing Strategy and Information: APA Practice Directorate

The American Psychological Association Practice Directorate has compiled a set of case studies from the literature on employer/corporate cost savings and the overall health cost savings that result when psychological services are incorporated into health benefits. Testing psychologists' awareness of these findings can aid in developing and marketing "products" that offer appropriate screening and assessment

189

services to clients via employers or other payors (insurers, medical facilities, bureaus of veterans affairs, and so on). The information in the following listings (APA, 1994, pp. 2–14) is reprinted with permission.

SIGNIFICANT SAVINGS AMONG CORPORATIONS

1. In 1989, BellSouth adopted a mental health benefit that encouraged employees to receive care in the least restrictive setting. BellSouth's bill for mental health dropped $6 million in the three following years.

2. Since 1989, McDonnell Douglas has used a mental health benefit that places no constraints on the type of treatment received. In the first year of utilization of this benefit, the company realized a 50% decrease in psychiatric inpatient admission costs, and per-capita mental health costs declined by 34%.

3. Between 1989 and 1992, the Civilian Health and Medical Program of the Uniformed Services (CHAMPUS) expanded its yearly outpatient psychiatric care expenditures from $81 million to $103 million. This decision to devote an additional $22 million to outpatient care resulted in a net savings of $200 million because of reduced psychiatric hospitalization.

4. In one year, after implementing a provider network that covered intermediary services and encouraged outpatient care, Chevron experienced a 21% decrease in psychiatric hospital admission costs.

5. First National Bank of Chicago saved 30% in mental health and substance abuse costs over four years as a result of implementing a mental health benefit that expanded the range of services covered and reimbursed outpatient costs at 85%.

6. In 1987, National Cash Register (NCR) began encouraging employees and their families to use a mental health plan that emphasized early intervention, access to a full range of care, and treatment in the least restrictive setting. NCR saved close to $300,000 in the first year alone. Projected savings for expanding the program are close to $2 million.

Medical Cost Offset

REDUCTION OF OVERALL HEALTH CARE COSTS
THROUGH MENTAL HEALTH INTERVENTION

1. Offset analysts studied medical and psychological histories of nearly 300 veterans from 1985 to 1987. Those receiving psychotherapy were compared to controls for psychological condition and medical utilization following an index period. Psychiatric patients whose pretreatment medical utilization was excessive showed a dramatic reduction in subsequent use of medical services after receiving abbreviated mental health treatment. These patients dropped from an average of 5.5 annual outpatient medical visits in 1985 to an average of 3.5 visits in 1987. Control groups, who received no psychotherapy, actually increased outpatient medical utilization. Subjects in all groups whose initial medical utilization levels were low or average maintained appropriate use of these services.

2. Research involving 20,000 Columbia Medical Plan participants (in Maryland) showed that untreated mentally ill patients increased their medical utilization by 61% during a one-year period. The mentally ill who received psychological treatment increased their medical expenditures by only 11%. The treated group's use of medical services was comparable to that of a comparison population with no diagnosable mental disorder, which averaged a 9% increase.

3. Modest psychological interventions have been shown to reduce hospital stays to approximately 1.5 days below control groups' average of 8.7 days.

4. Elderly patients who received mental health care averaged 12 fewer hospital days than a comparison group who were hospitalized for the same reasons but did not receive mental health care. This savings is important because older Americans are the fastest growing segment of the population. In 1992, people over the age of 50 accounted for less than 26% of the population. By 2050, this number will grow to more than 37%.

5. A study of a large population of Medicaid recipients and federal employees found that patients with chronic medical illnesses (e.g., diabetes and hypertension) lowered their medical costs 18% to 31% after receiving targeted psychological services.

6. Patients with more severe physical disorders can realize significant reductions in medical utilization if provided with mental health care. A study of the Georgia Medicaid population showed that patients who used inpatient services during a ten-quarter period spent $11,391. Outpatients spent a comparatively small $2,574 during the same period. Thus, patients undergoing surgery or other traumatic inpatient procedures have the highest potential to realize offset effects. (See also item 17.)

7. Other studies have shown that patients with functional limitations, including physical handicaps and debilitating physical ailments, show high potential for offset. The Rand Corporation designed a study involving nearly 4,500 subjects from six geographically diverse sites. Researchers assigned families to one of fourteen fee-for-service insurance plans that ranged in mental health coverage from free psychiatric care to almost no coverage. Each enrollee was tested for psychological and physical well-being using a battery of standard tests. The authors found that, in every category of mental health status (low, medium, or high functioning), those who had functional limitations (defined as physically caused impairment in ability to carry out the activities of daily living) used 50% to 100% more mental health services than those without such limitations. The study concluded that those with functional limitations due to poor health are high users of both medical and mental services. The high price of these subjects' health-care makes them excellent candidates for offset.

8. Diagnosing and treating patients with multiple personality disorder resulted in net savings of $84,900 per patient, in direct (medical) costs alone, during the first ten years following treatment.

9. Earlier diagnosis of patients with multiple personality disorder could save $250,000 per case in direct (medical) costs alone if the disorder is identified within the first year of the patient's utilization of medical care.

10. Borus and Olendzki (1985) showed that patients who are diagnosed with severe mental ailments but do not receive psychological treatment increase their medical utilization at significantly faster rates than those chronic patients who do receive treatment. These results indicate that unless the severely mentally ill enter the mental health system, they are likely to become voracious users of already

limited medical resources. These authors and other offset analysts suggest that, in the absence of appropriate psychiatric care, the cost to insurers and to the primary care system is astronomical.

11. Positive results take on even more significance when considering the prevalence of the four chronic diseases that afflict 40% of the American population: diabetes, ischemic heart disease, hypertension, or airway-respiratory conditions. Given the correct psychological intervention, many of these patients could limit their medical expenditures while simultaneously improving their mental health status—at virtually no cost.

12. Individuals who suffer from mental illness, and whose physical health problems are so severe that they are admitted for inpatient treatment, provide the greatest vehicle for saving physical health treatment dollars via the offset effect.

13. A National Institute of Mental Health (NIMH) study found that the cost of covering mental illness on the same basis as medical illness would be $6.5 billion. Spending this "extra" amount would save U.S. taxpayers $8.7 billion in indirect costs associated with untreated mental illnesses.

14. The Group Health Association found that patients receiving mental health counseling trimmed their nonpsychiatric usage by 30.7% and their use of laboratory and X-ray services by 29.8%.

15. When the Utah division of Kennecott Copper Corporation provided mental health counseling for employees, its hospital medical and surgical costs decreased 48.9%. The company's weekly claims costs dropped nearly 64.2%. In all, for every dollar spent on mental health care, the company saved $5.78.

16. A study of Kaiser Permanente patients who received psychotherapy showed the following decreases:

- 77.9% in the average length of stay in the hospital.
- 66.7% in frequency of hospitalizations.
- 48.6% in the number of prescriptions written.
- 48.6% in the number of physicians seen for office visits.
- 47.1% in physician office visits.
- 45.3% in emergency room visits.
- 31.2% in telephone contacts.

17. A study of the entire Georgia Medicaid population revealed substantial offset savings resulting from mental health treatments. Patients receiving inpatient physical health treatment in addition to their mental health treatment realized a cumulative savings of nearly $1,500 over a two-and-a-half-year period. The cost of the mental health intervention was entirely paid for (i.e., totally offset) by these savings. Patients were psychologically and physically healthier at essentially no charge. While not reaching total offset, patients who had no physical ailments requiring inpatient treatment but received mental health care still showed significant savings. This group, which contained both severe and less severe diagnoses, had medical health charges that were $296 to $392 lower than comparison samples during the study period.

18. A three-year study of over 10,000 Aetna beneficiaries showed that, after the initiation of mental health treatment, client medical costs dropped continuously over the next 36 months. The health costs of one mental health intervention group fell from $242 the year prior to treatment to $162 two years posttreatment. Other subject groups demonstrated similarly dramatic offset effects, leading the researchers to conclude that a decrease in total healthcare costs can be expected following mental health interventions *even when the cost of the intervention is included.*

19. Medicaid patients with drug and alcohol problems who received targeted psychological services reduced their subsequent medical costs by 15%. Those not receiving psychological assistance increased their medical costs by 90%.

20. A University of California study found that every $1.00 spent on drug and alcohol treatment saves society $11.54 in healthcare and criminal justice costs and lost productivity for business.

21. Scientists have found that failure to receive treatment for alcohol and substance abuse diagnoses can result in a very rapid escalation of individual medical costs. Cummings very recently concluded a study of Medicaid recipients in Hawaii. After a review of medical records, he found that patients diagnosed as chemically dependent who did not use mental health services increased their medical costs by 91% during the study period, compared to actual decreases in medical costs for treatment recipients. Some types of

intervention produced net decreases of approximately $514 per person in the first twelve months after treatment.

22. A study performed at the Columbia Medical Plan involved nearly 3,300 subjects who had experienced at least one psychiatric episode less than a year prior to the study. Researchers discovered a proportional relationship between the number of psychiatric visits and the number of medical visits, implying that persons most in need of intensive mental health services use inordinate amounts of medical resources.

23. Other researchers have proposed that mentally distressed persons are prime candidates for unnecessary surgical procedures, lab tests, and hospitalization. Instead of ameliorating psychological problems, these needless and expensive procedures may deteriorate the patient's psychological condition and cause a decrease in overall health.

24. Studies examining medical utilization before and after psychological treatment have shown that clients with large medical expenditures prior to treatment are most likely to show medical service reductions following treatment.

25. A study performed by Schlesinger et al. (1983) shows that outpatient mental health treatment is remarkably successful in reducing inpatient costs. Subjects included nearly 2,000 people diagnosed with one of four chronic diseases (diabetes, ischemic heart disease, hypertension, and airflow limitation disease). Over 700 patients received varying lengths of psychotherapy; the remainder served as a control sample. Researchers studied all groups for a three-year period, tracking medical expenditures and mental health status. Three years later, most intervention groups had medical costs that were between $284 and $309 lower than comparison groups. Offsets remained stable during the entire three-year study period. Twenty-five percent of the group receiving mental health realized a total offset, indicating that their treatments were essentially cost-free.

26. Jones and Vischi, reviewing the role of substance abuse treatment in medical cost offset, assessed 13 studies germane to alcohol/drug abuse interventions. The authors found that as much as 85% of medical expenditures could be reduced through treatment. The average reduction in medical utilization generated by mental health treatments was a sizable 20%. When the scope was broadened

to include sick days and accident benefits paid to employees, the median reduction doubled to 40%. In 1988 dollars, this median reduction represents $35.2 billion, nearly one-third the cost of the entire Medicare program. The review led researchers to conclude that strong evidence exists associating alcoholism treatment with subsequent reductions in medical utilization.

27. In his review of the offset literature, Shemo (1985–1986), a specialist on cost offset, found several indications that cost offsets increase over time. One of the most important reasons this occurs is that the treatment recipients continue to decrease their medical utilization, while seldom requiring any additional mental health services.

Lifestyle Enhancement, Wellness, and Prevention

Stair (1995) predicts that, by the year 2000, more employers will implement more preventive, wellness, health enhancement, and lifestyle-oriented programs. This forecast will likely be supported by the impact of capitated payment models. Capitation is actually one of the only models in which there is a fiscally based mechanism for funding prevention services. Although prevention has long been demonstrated to hold both humanitarian and economic benefits, funding programs are rare. Capitation should be a mode to provide funding in a more "real time" manner (i.e., benefits may manifest more quickly than just hoped-for offsets at some future point).

Stair notes the current most common corporate programs (and their frequency) related to wellness (1995, p. 12):

1. Smoking cessation programs (62%).
2. Regular blood pressure checks (50%).
3. Annual no-cost mammograms (49%).
4. Regular cholesterol checks (46%).
5. Wellness newsletters (45%).
6. Blood testing for illegal drugs (44%).
7. Prenatal education and care (43%).

8. Annual no-cost physical exam (43%).
9. Annual no-cost cervical cancer exam (37%).
10. Regular health checks (36%).

Future predictions suggest (Stair, 1995):

1. Smoking cessation programs (up 17% to 79%).
2. Wellness newsletters (up 25% to 70%).
3. Annual no-cost mammograms (up 19% to 68%).
4. Regular cholesterol checks (up 19% to 65%).
5. Regular blood pressure checks (up 12% to 62%).
6. Weight loss program (up 24% to 59%).
7. Prenatal education and care (up 15% to 58%).
8. Annual no-cost physical exam (up 14% to 57%).
9. Annual no-cost prostate exam (up 22% to 55%).
10. Annual no-cost cervical cancer exam (up 14% to 51%).

Of the areas addressed, the largest percentage gains lie within the psychological domain (e.g., wellness newsletters at 25% and weight loss programs at 24%). If the projections prove to be even somewhat accurate, it is important for psychologists to alter (if necessary) their population foci to include corporate contacts in order to help fill the current and projected needs of employers for their employees.

Some testing psychologists may need to gain additional training and expertise in lifestyle assessments and/or to develop screening and evaluation protocols for this new referral area. Also within the domain of psychologists are these additional needs noted by Stair (1995, p. 12):

1. Develop a means of measuring the success of the program.
2. Design a five-year plan to implement more preventive programs, beginning with those that will have the greatest and most immediate impact on healthcare spending.
3. Establish an employee communications program that emphasizes the importance of the program to both the employer and the employee.

Conclusion

Although medical cost offset issues and psychological assessment have a less direct connection than pairings in other contexts, these issues are important for psychologists who wish to expand their market share within the managed care environment. Testing psychologists who have an ability to coordinate educational and treatment resources, in addition to skill in testing and evaluation, will be able to design, market, and provide a comprehensive "turnkey" service package. A convenient, interrelated, non-piecemeal product that is accountable and cost-efficient in its service provision would hold great appeal to employers.

As the healthcare marketplace continues to rapidly evolve and change, psychologists must become more forthright in supporting the marked value and merit of psychological services as being on a par with other employee benefits, and just as necessary as medical, dental, vision, or other healthcare coverage. Psychologists should pursue resources for educating employers, employees, payors, benefit design managers, insurance consultants, and others, in the quantifiable, value-added aspects of psychological evaluation and care.

Recommended Readings

The following group of references is recommended for continuing applied clinical research. They also demonstrate the sheer (and often unrealized) vastness of the available studies. Psychological interventions can have a remarkable health and fiscal impact, especially through identification and referral/triage, on medical cost offset. (Full publication data are given in the References section, beginning on page 247.)

Armstrong, S. C., & Took, K. J. (1993).

Borus, J. F., & Olendzki, M. C. (1985).

Brody, D. S. (1980).

Cummings, N. A. (1990, February).

Cummings, N. A., Dorken, H., Pallak, M. S., & Henke, C. J. (1990).

Cummings, N. A., & Follette, W. T. (1968).

Dua, V., & Ross, C. (1993).

Fiedler, J. L., & Wight, J. B. (1989).

Franklin, J., & Williams, A. F. (1993).

Goodwin, F. K., & Moskowitz, J. (1993).

Hankin, J. R., Kessler, L. G., Goldberg, I. D., Steinwachs, D. M., & Starfield, B. H. (1983).

Holder, H. D., & Blose, J. O. (1987).

Inman, L. (1981).

Jencks, S. F. (1985).

Jones, K. (Ed.). (1979).

Kessler, L. G., Steinwachs, D. M., & Hankin, J. R. (1982).

Lechnyr, R. (1992).

Lechnyr, R. (1993).

Massad, P., West, A., & Friedman, M. (1990).

McGrady, B. S. (1986).

Mumford, E., Schlesinger, H., Glass, G., Patrick, C., & Cuerdon, T. (1984).

Nakamura, K., Tanaka, A., & Takano, T. (1993).

Schlesinger, H. J., Mumford, E., Gene, V., Glass, V., Patrick, C., & Shartstein, S. (1983).

Shemo, J. (1985–1986).

Shipley, R. H., Orleans, C. T., Wilbur, C. S., Piserchia, P., & McFadden, D. (1988).

Ware, J. E., Manning, W. G., Duan, N., Wells, K., & Newhouse, J. (1984).

Yates, B. T. (1984).

SECTION IV

MANAGING TESTING SERVICES IN THE NEW BEHAVIORAL FRONTIER

CHAPTER 9

Automating an Assessment Practice

WITHIN THE MANAGED care environment, or in any type of situation that demands cost and time savings along with an obligation to continue to provide high quality, automation can offer some solutions. Computers and communications technologies are becoming standards and norms, not options. Rarely, today, will a household have a rotary phone, black-and-white television, an AM-only radio, a manual typewriter, and an 8-track audio tape player. These technologies are not bad, but newer ones provide better quality and dependability, perhaps at less expense.

Ease of Use

A key factor in a technology's broad acceptance is its user-friendliness; that is, no matter how complex the task, the technology must make the instrument usable. Thus, a telephone, cellular phone, and beeper are all very easy to use, and they do not require the user to be conversant with fiber optics, cells, digitization, compression, bandwidth, or any other technological component. These design and application aspects will continue to drive the various office and industrial technologies that will be used in the future. Barrett and Vein (1995) realistically point out that computer use by practicing psychologists need not be intimidating. Productivity and quality enhancements can result from an automated psychology practice. This chapter broadly identifies various technological applications for testing psychologists.

Moore's Law posits that the capabilities of computer chips quadruple every three years. Thus, it is virtually impossible to author a chapter on technologies that is not providing some information that is a bit out of date, if not almost obsolete. With this in mind, this chapter will broadly canvass various automated domains that may be of use to testing psychologists' practices. Volumes of more detailed information are available, and anyone wishing to know more about a particular domain is encouraged to use the information provided herein to contact manufacturers, retailers, and publishers directly. This chapter's function is to give readers a resource for learning more about what technology exists and how it may prove to be helpful.

Office Hardware

Most testing psychologists have some basic office hardware: computer, printer, phone, answering system, photocopier. More advanced offices may have multiple computers linked together via a network. When any major capital expenditure is being considered, service needs, price, features, options, ease of use, and expandability should be purchase-decision factors. Many computers and peripherals now offer combined features. For example, some computers now can send and receive faxes, answer phones with voice mail, and dial phone numbers. Some printers are now capable of being serving additional duty as fax receivers, scanners, copiers, and file transfer devices.

PURCHASING DECISIONS

A fundamental question for any system change is: "Should we buy, build, or upgrade?" A consultant may help with the answer if one's practice is large (more than 15 clinicians, 3 or more office staff, and more than 500 procedures per month). Smaller offices may be able to use a retailer's advice and save the fee of an information services consultant. A good rule of thumb is to purchase a processor/modem that has the highest speed and is still affordable, along with as much disk storage as is possible within the budget, and three or more expansion slots (for upgradeability). The software applicable to psychological offices and clinical practices is abundant in IBM/compatible formats. Apple's Macintosh holds only approximately 10% of the personal computer market. Most users find that Microsoft's Windows™ is actually becoming the de facto standard. In this author's opinion, adoption of such a system avoids any likelihood of near-term obsolescence.

Because testing psychologists produce a large number of report documents, the printer purchased should be reliable, provide high-volume output, and have various font options and features. Laser printers are currently the best technology. Additional equipment purchases worth serious consideration include an uninterruptable power supply (which will also serve as a surge protector) and a data backup storage device. A wide variety of media are available for backup storage, such as quarter-inch and 8-mm cassette tape, digital audio tape (DAT) cassettes, PCMCIA cards, and writable CD optical storage. Costs vary widely, and although it is expensive, backup and electrical protection is a system "must."

Office Software

In a national survey of almost 600,000 physicians, conducted in 1995 by BMI Medical Information, Inc. (Arlington Heights, IL), surprisingly few medical doctors use computers in their practice. Their use of available computer functions was recorded as:

Access databases	6.6%
Patient billing	4.9
Insurer billing	4.1
Research	4.0
Record storage	2.8
Online claims processing	1.7
Issue prescriptions	0.2

TABLE 9.1
Core Office Practice Applications

	Windows	Macintosh
Database		
Lotus Approach 800-343-5415	Yes	No
Panorama II 2.1.3 800-966-7878	No	Yes
Integrated Software		
Claris Works 3.0 800-325-2747	Yes	Yes
Office Suites		
Microsoft Office 800-426-9400	Yes	Yes
Organizers		
Date Book & Touch Base Pro 4.0 800-833-6687	No	Yes
Day-Timer Organizer 1.0 800-859-6954	Yes	No
Reference		
Microsoft Bookshelf 1994 800-426-9400	Yes	Yes
Spreadsheets		
Microsoft Excel 5.0 800-426-9400	No	Yes
Word Perfect Quatro Pro 6.0 800-451-5151	Yes	No
Utilities		
Dashboard 2.0 800-533-0004	Yes	No
Norton Utilities 3.1 800-441-7234	No	Yes
Now Utilities 5.0 800-237-2078	No	Yes
PC Tools 2.0 800-964-6896	Yes	No
Word Processors		
Microsoft Word 6.0 800-426-9400	Yes	No
Communications		
Communications Software		
Crosstalk for Windows 2.2 800-348-3221	Yes	No
MicroPhone Pro 2.0.2 510-644-3232	No	Yes
Fax Software		
Fax Pro 1.5.1 800-268-6082	No	Yes
WinFax Pro 4.0 800-268-6082	Yes	No

TABLE 9.1 (Continued)

	Windows	Macintosh
Financial		
Accounting		
M.Y.O.B. 5.0 800-322-6962	No	Yes
Peachtree Accounting for		
Windows 3.0 800-247-3224	Yes	No
Personal Finance		
Quicken Deluxe for		
Windows 4.0 800-624-8742	Yes	No
Check Writer Pro		
For Macintosh 6.0 800-426-0854	No	Yes
DTP/Graphics (Business)		
Adobe IntelliPlan 2.0 800-833-6687	No	Yes
Visio 3.0 800-446-3335	Yes	No
Desktop Publishing (Midrange)		
Adobe Home Publisher 2.01 800-833-6687	No	Yes
Microsoft Publisher 2.0 800-426-9400	Yes	No
Presentation Graphics		
Astound 1.0 800-982-9888	No	Yes
Harvard Graphics for		
Windows 3.0 800-234-2500	Yes	No

It is not known how many psychologists currently use computers in their offices, but a future need of this technology is certain. Psychologists should be aware of the types of programs that are available and should examine them at a retailer or via a demonstration (demo) disk.

Table 9.1 gives novices a basis from which to explore. The listings are from *Home Office Computing*'s 1995 Editor's Picks Awards of Best Products (pp. 57–70). Manufacturers' names and phone numbers are provided.

Specialty Software

Specialty software is voluminous, and the number of vendors grows daily. An annual review, conducted by the American Health Care Association and published (typically, in March) in *Provider* magazine, is recommended for readers interested in learning more about systems that cover these areas in a general way:

Accounting.

Bar coding.

Case mix.

Data planning.

Dietary.

Minimum data set.

Payroll.

Personnel.

Pharmacy/Medication administration record.

Quality assurance.

Scheduling.

A recent issue of *Provider* listed an annotated group of approximately 70 software firms, with their contact data, available applications, and other important information. This is a good resource for larger-scale practice and facility needs. The listing is annually revised.

Behavior, Health, and Software Applications

There is a continuing exponential growth of developers, vendors, and products that are available to aid in psychodiagnostics, report writing, billing and office management, electronic charting, treatment planning, scheduling, pharmacology, decision support, practice management, outcomes, and more. (Turnkey integrated outcome packages are discussed in Chapter 5.)

As with the technologies previously discussed (and with all technologies in general), this listing may be outdated shortly after it is written. Also, in no way is this listing exhaustive, nor is it an endorsement of the companies or services listed. The list serves two primary purposes by providing (a) a sample of how broadbased and varied the available systems are, and (b) information that leads readers to helpful sources. (The following information was gathered from the most up-to-date promotional material available at the time of this writing.)

OFFICE MANAGEMENT SYSTEMS

The vendors and products listed in Table 9.2 provide systems that aid in practice management. Billing, office accounting, contract tracking, and, in some instances, utilization, quality, and outcomes management modules are among their offerings. Interested readers are encouraged to contact the source directly and request product information.

DIAGNOSTIC AND ASSESSMENT SOFTWARE AND VENDORS

The vendors listed in Table 9.3 provide a wide range of computer-administered or computer-scored software packages for psychological, learning, vocational, and other psychometric procedures and tests. (Readers may wish to review Chapter 4, which specifically notes various technological applications to testing practice.) System requirements and norms vary, so it is important for testing psychologists to fully evaluate any product prior to incorporating it into their professional practice.

Data Entry Methods

Data entry to various accounting or clinical systems is an important aspect of automated assistance. Some systems may be limited to only keyboard or manual entry; however, there are additional technologies to expedite data entry.

TABLE 9.2
Office Management Vendors and Products

Advanced Institutional Management Software	516-496-7700
Applied Computer Services	800-553-4055
Applied Computing Services	800-553-4055
Blue Cross/Blue Shield of Illinois—Electronic Data Interchanging	312-938-7697
Blumenthal Software, Inc.—Patient Billing System	607-724-0032
Boston Technologies, Inc.	609-692-4958
Brand Software—Therapist Helper	800-343-5737
Cambridge Software Labs—The Cure	508-352-8909
Cardiff Software—Teleform	619-259-6447
Client Billing System, Medical Information Systems, Inc.	800-424-0258
Clinistat	800-568-8266
CMHC Systems	800-434-CMHC
Costar Users Group—Costar	800-869-6301
DocuTrac, Inc.—Quick Doc QA	800-850-8510
Dr. Welford's Chart Notes—MedicaLogic	503-645-6442
Echo Management Group	800-635-8209
Health Communication Services	800-543-6711
Healthcare Automation, Inc.	401-272-6880
Hill Associates Healthcare Management Systems	603-898-3115
Interactive Health Systems, Inc.—Self-Discovery,	916-987-0516
Lavender & Wyatt Systems, Inc.—Human Services Management	800-846-5720
Med4th Systems—Care4th	414-963-1985
Medi Pay, Inc.	503-227-6491
Medical Records Institute, Therapeutic Learning Program, FOCUS	617-964-3923
Medicomp of Virginia—MedTrac	703-803-8080
Mental Health Benefits Modeling Program—APA Practice Directorate	202-336-5900
MHS—Shrink	800-456-3003
Mitchell & McCormick	404-939-6480
NCS Technology Division	800-347-7226
O.M.S.—Touched	800-588-6824

TABLE 9.2 (Continued)

Pacific Medsoft—Clinical Information Manager	916-583-2994
Patient Medical Records—S-O-A-P Patient Medical Record System	800-285-7627
Physician Micro Systems, Inc.—Practice Partner Patient Record	206-441-8490
Psych Community Access Sector Systems	206-467-9061
Q.D. Systems—Q.D. Clinical: Patient Medical Record System	510-525-8630
Rudd, Inc.—Sum Time	504-524-5752
Software Solutions, Inc.	513-932-6667
Sorg Associates—SATIS	207-866-7865
Strategic Decision Systems, Inc.—Connex	800-845-6505
Synergistic Office Solutions, Inc.—Case Manager/Office Manager	904-242-9100
Systems Plus, Inc.—Medical Manager	415-969-7047
Technicare Health Systems	216-493-0558
Therapist's Gene	503-297-2717
Tri-B Computer Systems	614-481-7517
UNI/CARE Systems, Inc.	813-954-3403
Velocity Healthcare Informatics	800-844-5648
Wallaby Software—MediView	800-883-4636
Well Being Systems Corporation	201-332-0434
Wenzel Group, Inc.	612-944-2699
John Wiley & Sons—Therascribe (Treatment Planning Software)	800-US-WILEY

OPTICAL MARK RECOGNITION

Optical mark recognition (OMR) is a familiar technology to most testing psychologists. OMR uses a scanner that "reads" circles (also known as bubbles) that are filled in with dark pencil by the respondent. Scannable answer sheets exist for many objective tests (e.g., MMPI-2, CPI, and 16PF). A testing psychologist or trained staff person would "run" the sheet through the scanner, and this process inputs the patient's responses into a database or scoring system in the computer. OMR technology is robust and has few scanning-related errors. This is

TABLE 9.3
Software Vendors

American Guidance Service	800-328-2560
Anderson Publishing Co.	800-582-7295
Behaviordyne, Inc.	800-627-2673
Caldwell Report	213-478-3133
CFKR Career Materials, Inc.	800-525-5626
Clinical Psychometric Research, Inc.	800-245-0277
Computerized Psychological Diagnostics, Inc.	714-833-7931
Consulting Psychologists Press	800-624-1765
DLM Technical Resources	800-527-4747
Educational Technologies, Inc.	800-882-4384
Hilson Research, Inc.	718-805-0063
IPAT	800-225-4728
Life Science Associated	516-472-2111
London House/SRA	800-221-8378
Mental Health Connections, Inc.	800-788-4743
Metri Tech	800-747-4868
Multi-Health Systems, Inc.	800-456-3003
NCS Assessments—MicroTest Q	800-627-7271
New Standards, Inc.	612-690-1002
NiJo Software	914-472-6265
PAR, Inc.	800-331TEST
Pre-Ed, Inc.	512-451-3246
Precision People, Inc.	800-338-0710
Preventive Measures, Inc.	913-842-5078
Psych Support Systems	800-776-0519
Psychological Corporation	800-228-0752
Psychological Testing Service	517-631-9463
Psychologics	800-528-6244
Psychologistics, Inc.	407-259-7811
Psychometric Software, Inc.	800-882-9811
Psytex Services	800-392-5454
Reason House	301-321-7270
Roche Diagnostic Systems—Test Trakk	800-526-1247
SASSI Institute	800-726-0526
Sigma Assessment Systems, Inc.	800-265-1285
21st Century Assessment	800-374-2100
Upjohn Company—SDDS-PC	616-323-4000
Vocational Research Institute	800-874-5387
Western Psychological Service	800-648-8857

a key point in the test scoring; OMR is superior to optical character recognition.

OPTICAL CHARACTER RECOGNITION

Optical character recognition (OCR) technology allows for limited entry of data that are scanned via an OCR scanner. OCR scanners may be handheld or may resemble a small photocopy bed (known as a flat-bed scanner). With some software programs, printed handwriting can be "read" as well as darkened circles (similar to OMR). This software is less accurate in its recognition capabilities compared to OMR, but OMR cannot translate printed input. (Some software captures images, such as graphics or photos. This is helpful for electronic charts with patient's photos, or for a newsletter production.) Programs such as Teleform™ (from Cardiff, Inc.) allow testing psychologists to develop their own data collection tools for quick input of data into a database.

VOICE RECOGNITION SOFTWARE

Current technology in the area of voice or speech recognition software is rapidly evolving. Many existing systems allow certain commands to be voice-entered. Most testing psychologists will find speech-to-text transcription programs of marked benefit in dictating reports and clinical notes directly to electronic media and on to print. These programs are not flawless, but they can aid in accelerating report production if one does not type too well. The technology often requires laborious training of both the user and the software. Method, speed, articulation, and modulation of one's voice can be frustrating and time-consuming as the program "learns." Prices typically vary, according to capability and range, from around $200 to $2,500. Some contacts are:

Dragon Systems—Dragon Dictate Systems	617-965-5200
Kurzweil Voice for Windows v 1.0	617-893-5151
Power Secretary v 1.1.1	800-443-7077
Scribe v 2.0	215-747-5035

Computer-Assisted Therapy

Some testing psychologists initially feared that the computerization of psychological tests would result in obsolescence of the specialty. This did not occur. Similar fears, however, manifested some years ago with a program (now considered primitive) called ELIZA (Weizenbaum, 1966). This was basically an artificial intelligence program (of sorts) that reflected back a "patient's" input via a Rogerian style. It was an experiment of technology more than an instrument of psychotherapy.

Today, technological advances have resulted in some managed care companies actually offering patients the option of computer-administered therapy or human-administered therapy. Gould (1994) has developed the Therapeutic Learning Program (TLP) as an aid to support and reinforce the counselor's sessions. TLP is interactive with the patient.

Selmi, Klein, Griest, Sorrell, and Erdman (1990) evaluated an earlier product (Selmi, 1983) that utilized a cognitive-behavioral program for treating depression within an artificial intelligence framework. Colby and Colby (1992) have available a similar type of system known as *Overcoming Depression 2.0*. Stutske, Netzhamer, and Stout (in press) evaluated both programs, along with a computer cohort control group and a noncomputer cohort control group. The population was depressed inpatients receiving "traditional" therapies. The findings indicated that both experiential groups (those using the computer artificial intelligence programs) had decreased in depression to a degree that significantly differed from that of noncomputer cohort controls. General findings indicate some promise in the use of such artificial intelligence software as an aid in treatment. Kaiser Permanente's Department of Psychiatry is experimenting with virtual reality technology in treating phobias. Results are promising, and further research to investigate "Virtual Therapy" (Lamson, 1995) is planned.

Computer Curriculum Corporation (800-227-8324) has developed a multimedia, interactive CD-ROM called "Choosing Success" (Kline, 1995). Albeit not an interactive therapy program per se, it is unique in its construction and in its frank examination of family problems, gang violence, suicide, dating stresses, and other realistic concerns of adolescents today. It provides the following framework for dealing with such problems:

1. Define the *Challenge*.
2. Convey *Information*.
3. Identify the *Options*.
4. Choose an *Action*.
5. Verify the *Outcome*.

At this point, it is only available to schools as a component of an educational package, but more programs will likely be developed and available for other clinical and educational applications.

Information Services

The Internet is an exponentially expanding resource for anyone with a computer, modem, phone line, and access software. Among the companies that provide access services are Netcom, Prodigy, CompuServe, America Online, Genie, Delphi, and others. Many companies provide their software for low or no cost, but service and online costs can vary a great deal. Systems for access are becoming more user-friendly and graphically interfaced. A number of guides, books, articles, and entire magazines are devoted to the Internet. Services such as the World Wide Web, Archie, Veronica, Jughead, news groups, chat lines, bulletin boards, e-mail, and more are common to most systems. New users (referred to as "newbies" in the Internet vernacular) need not be intimidated, but should expect to be a little overwhelmed during their first few log-ons.

Most users of any online service will wish to have a modem that processes at least at a 9,600-baud rate (or bits per second, BPS). As with most devices, more (or in this instance, *faster*) is better. Thus, 14.4 (14,000 BPS) or 28.8 modems are preferred. The faster a modem operates, the faster information is delivered to one's computer. As hypertext and graphical interfaces become more popular on the Internet, faster communications will become a must. (If files are transferred via modem, there is always the risk of "catching a virus." It is a good practice to run a virus-check program episodically to act as a safeguard.)

Most psychologists will soon have e-mail addresses, just as they have evolved to beepers, answering machines, and faxes. Growth and increasingly user-friendly interfaces will ensure this. Growth in users is paralleled by growth in services offered. Below is a very brief sample of available offerings that are likely to be of interest to testing psychologists. Many other services are available, and the number is increasing almost daily.

Schoech and Smith (1995, pp. 25, 27) have provided the following bulletin boards (BBS) and Internet sites:

Behavioral Healthcare-Oriented BBS

	Location	BBS Phone
National Association of Social Workers	New Mexico	505-646-2868
Dissociation Net	Albany, NY	518-462-6134
Shrink Tank	California	408-257-8131
Testing Station	Indiana	317-846-8917
Statistics BBS	Kansas	316-687-0578
Bureau of Health Professions	Silver Spring, MD	301-443-5913

CONFERENCES ON THE INTERNET

Most printed lists of conferences on the Internet are outdated. However, one can quickly search for conferences on any topic by sending a message to listserv@vm1.nodak.edu. In the body of the message, type: LIST GLOBAL/[keyword]. To subscribe to any listserv, send a message to: listserv@listserv.net with the following command in the text (not the subject) of the message: SUBSCRIBE [listname]. Replace "listname" with the networkwide ID name in the first column of Table 9.4.

American Psychological Association (APA) Division 12 (Clinical Psychology) member access (DIV12NET) is maintained

216

TABLE 9.4
Listserv Subscriber Addresses

Networkwide ID	Full Address	List Description
APASD-L	APASD-L@VTVM1.BITNET	APA Research Psychology Network
COMPSY-L	COMPSY-L@UIUCVMD.BITNET	Midwest Forum for Community/Ecological Psychology
COUNPSY	COUNPSY@UGA.BITNET	Counseling psychology practice and science
EAWPO-L	EAWPO-L@HEARN.BITNET	European Association of Work/Organizational Psychology
IOOB-L	IOOBF-L@UGA.BITNET	Industrial psychology
IOOBF-L	IOBBF-L@UGA.BITNET	Industrial Psychology Forum
LEARN-L	LEARN-L@MIZZOU1.BITNET	Cognitive psychology and conditions for learning
MENTOR	MENTOR@INDYCMS.BITNET	Psychology b104 computer communications
PSYCH	PSYCH@INDYCMS.BITNET	Psychology department
PSYSTS-L	PSYSTS-L@MIZZOU1.BITNET	Psychology statistics discussion
VIRTPSY	VIRTPSY@SJUVM.BITNET	SJU virtual psychology list

by Ian Pitchford (without cost). Send an e-mail message to MAILBASE@MAILBASE.ac.uk with the message:

Join div12net [your first name last name]

For psychiatry, use:

Join psychiatry [your first name last name]

For psychiatry resources, use:

Join psychiatry-resources [your first name last name]

Division 12's GEROPSYCH (Section 2's Clinical Gero Psychology) net information is available via Barry Edelstein at u21b@wvnvm. wvnet.edu. The APA also has a website at http:\\www.apa.com. CompuServe offers a forum for medical computing, and others will likely evolve.

Of final note, the National Library of Medicine (NLM) maintains a searchable database of 3,700 medical journals via the online service of Medical Literature Analysis and Retrieval System (MEDLARS). One of the key components of MEDLARS is MEDLINE. It maintains over 7 million citations to biomedical articles and is searched, on the average, over 18,000 times daily (Murphy, 1995). MEDLINE is accessed via a very user-friendly package called "Grateful Med." Table 9.5 provides a history of the MEDLINE databases.

Grateful Med is available at 800-423-9255. It costs $29.95 pre-paid and the search charge is $18/hour.

Videoconferencing

Psychologists may find themselves attending more "virtual" meetings and conferences as the use of computers increases. Satellite downlinks have been frequently used to "telecast" some meetings and events. Often, the only interaction with such links is via telephone calling of questions or responses to the source or studio of the satellite feed. Desktop systems on individual computer platforms can be used for

TABLE 9.5
MEDLINE Databases

AIDSDRUGS. A description of substances being tested in AIDS-related trials.

AIDSLINE (AIDS information onLINE). References to recent literature on AIDS and related topics.

AIDSTRIALS (AIDS clinical TRIALS).

AVLINE (Audio-Visuals onLINE).

BIOETHICSLINE (BIOETHICS onLINE).

CANCERLIT (CANCER LITerature).

CATLINE (CATalog onLINE). Bibliographic record of books related to health and medicine.

CCRIS (Chemical Carcinogenesis Research Information System).

CHEMID (CHEMical IDentification).

CHEMLINE (CHEMical dictionary onLINE).

DIRLINE (Directory of Information Resources onLINE). A listing of organizations that provide medical and health-related information services electronically.

HEALTH. Health planning and administration.

HSDB (Hazardous Substances Data Bank).

HSTAR (Health Service/Technology Assessment Research).

MEDLINE (MEDlars onLINE). The National Library of Medicine's premier bibliographic database; covers the fields of medicine, nursing, dentistry, veterinary medicine, and the preclinical sciences.

PDQ (Physician Data Query). Information on advances in cancer treatment and clinical trials.

RTECS (Registry of Toxic Effects of Chemical Substances).

SDILINE (Selective Dissemination of Information onLINE). References to biomedicine topics.

SERLINE (SERials onLINE). Biomedical serial titles.

TOXLINE (TOXicology information onLINE).

TOXLIT (TOXicology LITerature from special sources). Covers toxicological, pharmacological, biochemical, and physiological effects of drugs and other chemicals.

TRI (Toxic Chemical Release Inventory). A series.

TRIFACTS (Toxic Chemical Release Inventory FACT Sheet).

---

access. The industry is expected to reach $10.8 billion by 1997. Systems can begin as low as $3,500 but, with add-ons and dedicated lines, costs can quickly top $500,000.

Collaborative screen-sharing allows users at various sites to simultaneously view the same screen images. No other type of viewing (such as faces during videoconferencing) is allowed. The systems are much less expensive and easy to use. They require only a standard computer with supporting software, a modem, and a standard phone line. Telephone conferencing has improved beyond traditional speaker-phone capabilities. Systems today provide CD-quality sound along with bidirectional, simultaneous conversations (without bothersome blankouts). Convenient, time-saving conferencing, where a discussion can be clearly communicated, is possible at low cost.

Groupware programs (such as the popular Lotus Notes) allow for easy e-mail communication between users, without a need for Internet connections or changes beyond the initial software purchase and telephone line time. These programs are a primary aid in rapid communications with others, no matter where they are located.

The Mobile Psychologist and the Virtual Office

Today, testing psychologists are mobile psychologists—they work on site at hospitals, medical centers, physicians' offices, schools, corporations, incarceration facilities, and various other evaluation venues. The technologies of beepers, cellular phones, and notebook computers are currently very helpful in keeping psychologists in contact with their offices and referral sources. With the addition of faxes and voice mail paging/forwarding, the "virtual office" concept is complete.

PORTABLE COMPUTERS

Managed care constraints will likely cause many psychologists to become even more mobile in practice expansion and related consultant travel. As for computers, buyers have options of notebooks (currently selling for around $1,500+ with basic features), subnotebooks (smaller, less functional versions of notebooks, typically priced at less than $1,000), and power notebooks (costing $2,500+, with better graphics capabilities and other features). Many power notebooks, especially those with CD-ROM devices, are power tools for professional presentations, lectures, and marketing contacts, when coupled with projection devices or linked into a bank of color monitors.

MOBILE PHONES

Cellular phones are gaining in popularity as they drop in price and gain increased features. Not all geographic areas offer "cell sites," but this will change in time. Functions can be confusing and actually offer little value added; they include speed dialing, 100 alphanumeric memory, last 20 numbers called, call waiting, call restriction, pager functions, multiple call timers, multiple varied locks, signal strength, battery strength, and so on. The key issue is service cost. Many packages offer lower rates that aid in cost control. (Consumer-psychologists are warned to read the fine print before buying a phone that comes with an air-time service contract.)

There are interfaces that allow for linkage between cellular phones and notebook computers. This combination provides the opportunity to use cellular service (albeit expensive) to fax, e-mail, send/receive alphanumeric pages, or connect to the Internet via a mobile, wireless location.

SMART PAGERS

Pagers have been developed that offer global coverage not just of phone numbers but also of alphanumeric messages, information services, stock quotes, and other information. Two-way pagers now exist.

RECORDING DEVICES

Microcassette recorders have long been used by testing psychologists to record thoughts and dictate reports. These devices have gotten smaller and new features have been added. Digital audio tapes (DATs) that are the size of postage stamps have been available in Japan since 1993. Digital technology "cards" are inexpensive recorders, but they store only a limited amount of information and would not currently be appropriate for dictation.

Personal Digital Assistants

Many manufacturers are exploring (or have already developed) personal digital assistants (PDAs). Apple Computers has the Newton, Sony has Magic Link, and Motorola has the Envoy. Current PDAs are keyboardless, highly portable, and very user-friendly. They serve the multiple functions of telecommunications (fax, pager, phone, e-mail), organization (scheduling, planning, calendar, addresses, reminders), writing and drawing (sketching, drafts, animation, sound), and desktop functions (filing, time, calculation, Rolodex). Similar to voice recognition technology's limitations, handwriting recognition is limited and requires "training," but it is likely to improve.

Most PDAs also link to peripherals such as keyboard add-ons, printers, PCMCIA cards, and other desktop and notebook computers. Various other software applications can be loaded or are preprogrammed, such as accounting spreadsheets, spelling checkers, games, and online services. These technologies are likely to continue to develop and advance. Testing psychologists may consider their use in patient scheduling and practice management.

Future projections have PDAs doing less computer activity and more communication functions. Carnegie Mellon University is developing wearable computers, and Timex already has a watch that interfaces with the owner's computer to download schedule information (Ross, 1995). Ross notes that future PDAs will become faster, smaller, and lighter; will respond to voice commands; and will incorporate wireless video phone communications. Other forecasts suggest that they will be part of clothing or worn as accessories. Their interfaces will incorporate a "personality," and some devices may be purchased not just for features but for the "attitude" of the machine.

Additional Resources

Software information is available from a number of sources. The following listing represents a heterogeneous mix of publications that are of interest to testing psychologists:

APA Monitor
American Psychiatric Association
750 First Street
Washington, DC 20002

Behavioral Health Management
Mediquest Communications, Inc.
629 Euclid Avenue, Suite 500
Cleveland, OH 44114

Behavioral Healthcare Tomorrow
4370 Alpine Road, Suite 108
. Portola Valley, CA 94028

Computers in Mental Health: A Selected Bibliography
(1992; D. W. Viewes and J. L. Hedlund)
University of Missouri
Department of Psychiatry
5247 Fyler Avenue
St. Louis, MO 63139

Computer Use in Psychology: A Directory of Software, 3rd edition
(1992; M. L. Stoloff & J. V. Couch, Eds.)
American Psychiatric Association, Inc.
Order Department
P. O. Box 2710
Hyattsville, MD 20784

Medical Software Reviews
462 Second Street
Brooklyn, NY 11215-2503

Open Minds
44 South Franklin Street
Gettysburg, PA 17325

Physicians and Computers
Moorehead Publications, Inc.
810 S. Waukegan Road, Suite 200
Lake Forest, IL 60045

Behavioral Health Treatment
Manisses Communications Group, Inc.
208 Governor Street
Providence, RI 02906-0757

Software News
Mental Health Connections, Inc.
21 Blossom Street
Lexington, MA 02173

Conclusion

What will the future hold? Matarazzo (1992) forecasts that intelligence testing in the future will be biological, not psychological. Imaging technologies of PET, MRI, CAT, SPECT, and even imaged EEGs will likely start to be applied to psychiatric diagnoses. Computers will be more user-friendly for patients and psychologists. Considering testing psychology's basis in science, advancements in testing applications should be quite exciting. Virtual reality technology, computer-aided testing, and multimedia and interactive systems will have further applications to testing and clinical practice.

Use of such tools will aid in providing higher-quality services within managed care or in any type of payor environment. It is important for psychologists to not fear the current technologies, as they will likely come to embrace the future's technological advances.

APPENDIX

---

*Characteristics of Products
Available for Assessment*

Product	Format	Cost	Source
Alcohol Use Inventory (AUI)	Paper and pencil Computer Self-report	$55.00 starter package	National Computer Systems, Inc. 5605 Green Circle Drive Minnetonka, MN 55343 800-627-7271
Behavior and Symptom Identification Scale (BASIS)	Paper and pencil	Permission of authors; no fee	Eisen, S., Grob, M., & Klein, A. (1986). BASIS: The development of a self-report measure for psychiatric evaluation. *The Psychiatric Hospital, 6,* 165–171.
Brief Symptom Index (BSI)	Paper and pencil Computer Cassette	$2.35 each (500 minimum)	National Computer Systems, Inc. 5605 Green Circle Drive Minnetonka, MN 55343 800-627-7271
Child & Adolescent Functional Assessment Scale	Paper and pencil		Dr. Kay Hodges 2140 Earhart Road Ann Arbor, MI 48105 313-769-9725

Characteristics of Products Available for Assessment

Capabilities	Advantages	Disadvantages
Behavior, attitudes, symptom identification Primary Scales: • Benefits • Consequences • Styles • Concerns & acknowledgments Second-Order Factor Scales General Alcohol Involvement Scale	Adult and adolescent population Results coordinated with DSM classification system Treatment recommendations Suggestions for further evaluation	Specific to alcohol-related presenting problems
Function assessment Diagnostic group discrimination	Self-report	Limited to psychiatric inpatient population
Psychological symptom pattern measurement Severity of illness ratings: • Global Severity Index • Symptom Distress Index • Symptom Total Symptom dimensions • Anxiety • Interpersonal sensitivity • Phobic anxiety • Depression • Paranoid ideation • Somatization • Hostility • Obsessive-compulsive • Psychoticism	13 years and older medical and psychiatric population Reliability detects changes in patient's symptoms and severity of course of treatment Can be integrated within software system with other measures (e.g., HSQ) from NCS	
Assesses child and adolescent populations' level of functioning		Limited to child and adolescent populations

(continued)

Product	Format	Cost	Source
Child Behavior Checklist and Youth Self-Report	Paper and pencil		University Associates in Psychiatry c/o Child Behavior Checklist One South Prospect Street Burlington, VT 05401 802-656-8313 (voice) 802-656-2602 (fax)
Community Adaptation Schedule			Burns, A., & Roen, S. (1967) Social roles and adaptation to the community. *Community Mental Health Journal, 3*, 153–158.
Coping Resources Inventory (B)	Paper and pencil Hand-scored Computer-scored	$21.00; 25 booklets $54.00; 10 prepared answer sheets—mailin scoring $40.00; handscoring keys $26.00; 25 answer sheets	Consulting Psychologists Press, Inc. 3803 East Bayshore Road P.O. Box 10096 Palo Alto, CA 94303 800-624-1765

Capabilities	Advantages	Disadvantages
Assesses child and adolescent behavior functioning and problems		Limited to children and adolescent populations
Social/community functioning measurement Occupational/school functioning measurement Assesses: • Social life • Substance abuse • "Law" trouble • Affect • Mood • Family relationship • Household responsibility • Recreation • General "happiness"	Broad-based measure	217 items Does not include specific psychiatric symptoms
Measures resources inherent in people that facilitate stress management	Ten-minute administration Self-report Identifies individuals at high risk for stress-related problems Age: middle school to adults	

(continued)

Product	Format	Cost	Source
Derogatis Psychiatric Rating Scale (DPRS)	Paper and pencil Clinician rating form	$69.50 per 50	National Computer Systems, Inc. 5605 Green Circle Drive Minnetonka, MN 55343 800-627-7271
Ellsworth Adjustment and Adaptation Profiles (B)	Paper and pencil	$15.00/package of 25 per each of 4 profiles	Consulting Psychologists Press, Inc. 3803 East Bayshore Road P.O. Box 10096 Palo Alto, CA 94303 800-624-1765

Characteristics of Products Available for Assessment

Capabilities	Advantages	Disadvantages
Initial evaluation of patient Outcomes evaluation of patient Provides nine primary system dimension scales: • Somatization • Depression • Anxiety • Hostility • Psychoticism • Obsessive-compulsive • Interpersonal sensitivity • Phobic anxiety • Paranoid ideation Global Pathology Index (GPI) Provides eight additional dimensional scales: • Excitement • Euphoria • Hysterical • Abjection/disinterest • Sleep disturbance • Psychomotor retardation • Conceptual behavior dysfunction • Disorientation	Adult and adolescent population usage Administration time: 2 to 5 minutes	Used in conjunction with SCL-90-R or BSI
Measures adjustment to the community Multiple forms: • Child & Adolescent Adjustment Profile (CAAP)—measures peer relations, dependency, hostility, productivity, withdrawal		

(continued)

Product	Format	Cost	Source
FACES III	Paper and pencil		Family Social Science Department University of Minnesota 290 McNeal Hall 1985 Beuford Avenue St. Paul, MN 55108 612-628-7250
Geriatric Depression Scale (geriatric population)	Paper and pencil		Yesavage, J., Brink, T., Rose, T., Lum, O., Huang, O., Adey, V., & Leirer, V. (1983). Development and validation of a geriatric depression

Characteristics of Products Available for Assessment

Capabilities	Advantages	Disadvantages
• Adult Personal Adjustment and Role Skills (APARS)—measures close relations, alienation-depression, anxiety, confusion, ETOH/drug use, house activity, child relations, employment; filled out by someone close to the patient • Profile of Adaptation to Life—Clinical (PAL-C)—self-report; measures negative emotions, well-being, income management, physical symptoms, ETOH/drug use, close relations, child relations • Profile of Adaptation to Life—Holistic (PAL-H)—self-report; measures social activity, self-activity, nutrition, exercise, personal growth, spiritual awareness		
Assesses child and adolescent populations' level of functioning		Limited to child and adolescent populations
Assessment of depression in geriatric populations	Ease of use	Limited to geriatric populations

(continued)

Product	Format	Cost	Source
			screening scale: A preliminary report. *Journal of Psychiatric Research, 17,* 37–49. *or* Yesavage, J. (1988). Geriatric Depression Scale. *Psychopharmacology Bulletin, 24*(4), 709–711.
Global Assessment of Functioning [Revision of the Global Assessment Scale, Endicott et al. (1976)]	Paper and pencil Therapist rating	$0	American Psychiatric Association. (1994). *Diagnostic and Statistical Manual of Mental Disorders* (4th ed.). Washington, DC: Author.
Global Assessment Scale	Paper and pencil Therapist rating	$0	Endicott, I., Spitzer, R., Fleiss, J., & Cohen, J. (1976). The Global Assessment Scale. *Archives of General Psychiatry, 33,* 766–771.
Health Plan Employee Data and Information Sheet (HEDIS-25)	Chart review scoring schema	Varies widely as a function of who purchaser is	National Committee for Quality Assurance (NCQA) 1350 New York Avenue, N.W., Suite 700 Washington, DC 20005 202-662-8610
Index of Activities of Daily Living (ADL)—geriatric population	Paper and pencil		Katz, S., Ford, R., Moskowitz, R., Jackson, B., & Jaffe, M. (1963). Studies of illness in the aged. The index of ADL:

Capabilities	Advantages	Disadvantages
Procedure for measuring overall severity of psychiatric disturbance	Easy to use Quick	Unsophisticated 10-interval scoring system is only information provided; therefore, limited and subjectively imprecise
Procedure for measuring overall severity of psychiatric disturbance	Easy to use Quick	Unsophisticated 10-interval scoring system is only information provided; therefore, limited and subjectively imprecise
760 performance measures Performance information report: • Quality • Utilization • Finance • Enrollee access • Enrollee satisfaction	Purchasers can better assess value of healthcare dollar Holds healthcare plans accountable for their performance	May not apply well to behavioral health field Cost Time/labor
General quality-of-life measurement Determines impact of disease/disability on function and ability to perform role activities in everyday life	Used widely in determining independence factors of the geriatric population	Does not make suggestions toward the well end of the quality-of-life continuum Would not work well to survey noninstitutionalized population

(continued)

235

Product	Format	Cost	Source
			A standardized measure of biological and psychosocial function. *Journal of the American Medical Association, 185,* 914–919.
Inventory of Suicide Orientation— 30 (ISO-30): • *30 items* • *10-minute administration* • *Patient management suggestions*	Paper and pencil Computer	$30.00 starter package $13.00 reorder (per 25)	National Computer Systems, Inc. 5605 Green Circle Drive Minnetonka, MN 55343 800-627-7271
Lawton/Brody Instrumental ADL Scale	Paper and pencil		Lawton, M., & Brody, E. (1969). Assessment of older people: Self-maintaining and instrumental activities of daily living. *Gerontologist, 9,* 179–186. *or* Lawton, M., & Brody, E. (1988). Instrumental activities of daily living (IADL). *Psychopharmacology Bulletin, 24*(4), 785–791.
Mini Mental State Examination	Paper and pencil		Folstein, J., Folstein, S., & McHugh, P. (1975). Mini-mental state: A practical method for grading the cognitive state of patients for the clinician. *Journal of Psychiatric Research, 12,* 189–198. *or*

Characteristics of Products Available for Assessment

Capabilities	Advantages	Disadvantages
Suicide risk classification Hopelessness measurement Suicide ideation measurement		Applies to adolescent population only
General quality-of-life measurement Instrumental life activities measurement	Wide use	
Assessment and rating of cognitive status of geriatric populations	Ease of training and use	Limited to geriatric populations

(continued)

Product	Format	Cost	Source
			Cockrell, J., & Folstein, M. (1988). Mini-Mental State Examination. *Psychopharmacology Bulletin, 24*(4), 689–692.
Personality and Social Network Adjustment Scale	Paper and pencil		Clark, A. (1968). The Personality and Social Network Adjustment Scale: Its use in evaluation of treatment in a therapeutic community. *Human Relations, 21*, 85–95.
Problem-Solving Inventory (B)	Individual administration Group administration	$18.75 for 25 $7.50; scoring key $18.00; manual	Consulting Psychologists Press, Inc. 3803 East Bayshore Road P.O. Box 10096 Palo Alto, CA 94303 800-624-1765
Progress Evaluation Scales	Paper and pencil		Ihilevich, D. (1982). *Evaluating mental health progress: The Progress Evaluation Scales.* Lexington, MA: Lexington Books.
Quality of Life Enjoyment and Satisfaction Questionnaire	Paper and pencil Self-report		Endicott, J., Nee, J., Harrison, W., & Blumenthal, R. (1993). Quality of Life Enjoyment and Satisfaction Questionnaire: A new measure. *Psychopharmacology Bulletin, 29*, 321–326.

Characteristics of Products Available for Assessment

Capabilities	Advantages	Disadvantages
Social/community functioning measurement Occupational/school functioning measurement Assesses: • Family relationship • Substance abuse • "Law" trouble • Affect • Mood • Social life • Household responsibility • Recreation • General "happiness"	17 items	
Problem-solving and coping measurements Self-appraisal of problem-solving process Cognitive, affective, behavioral variable prediction	16 years and older 10-minute administration	
Social/community functioning measurement Occupational/school functioning measurement	7 items	
Measures degree of enjoyment and satisfaction by patients in daily functioning areas Overall severity of illness measurement	Assesses quality of life 93 items 8 summary scales Reliable for depressed outpatients (limited testing) Valid for depressed outpatients (limited testing)	Questionnaire broad based reliability and validity Age range

(continued)

Product	Format	Cost	Source
Quality of Life Inventory (QOLI)	Paper and pencil Computer	$40.00 package	National Computer Systems, Inc. 5605 Green Circle Drive Minnetonka, MN 55343 800-627-7271
Recovery Attitude and Treatment Evaluator (RAATE)	Paper and pencil Computer-scored	$137.50; hand-scoring templates	New Standards, Inc. 1080 Montreal Avenue, Suite 300 St. Paul, MN 55116 800-755-6299
Self-Assessment Guide	Paper and pencil		Willer, B., & Biggin, P. (1976). Comparison of rehospitalized and nonhospitalized psychiatric patients on community adjustment: Self-assessment guide. *Psychiatry, 39,* 239–244.

Characteristics of Products Available for Assessment

Capabilities	Advantages	Disadvantages
Develops effective treatment programs Identifies health problem risk Tracks treatment progress (administered pre- and posttreatment)	5-minute administration High reliability High validity Sensitive to change Helps establish comparative efficacy of treatments or service delivery systems (e.g., managed care) Non-health-related/personal health settings usage	
Continuing care measurement Appropriate treatment placement measurement Indicates: • Resistance to treatment • Biomedical problems • Social/family environmental status •Resistance to continual care •Psychiatric problem activity	Good test/retest reliability Easy to administer Easy to score 94 items	Administration time: 30 to 45 minutes
Social/community functioning measurement Occupational/school functioning measurement Assesses: • Family relationship • Substance abuse • "Law" trouble • Affect • Mood • Social life • Household responsibility • Recreation • General "happiness"	55 items	

(continued)

Product	Format	Cost	Source
Sickness Impact Profile (SIP)	Paper and pencil		Greenfield, S. (1991). The use of outcomes in medical practice applications of two medical outcomes studies. In J. Couch (Ed.), *Health care quality management for the 21st century.* Tampa, FL: American College of Physician Executives.
Social Adjustment Scale (SAS)			Weissman, M., & Bothwell, S. (1976). Assessment of social adjustment by patient self-report. *Archives of General Psychiatry, 33,* 1111–1115.
Symptom Checklist— 90 Analogue	Observer rating format	$30.00 per 100	National Computer Systems, Inc. 5605 Green Circle Drive Minnetonka, MN 55343 800-627-7271

Capabilities	Advantages	Disadvantages
Quality-of-life measure describing effect of sickness on behavioral function 136 items Independent index Physical index Psychosocial index	Can be used with many cultural subgroups Applicable to any disease/disability group	
Social/community functioning measurement Occupational/school functioning measurement Assesses: • Family relationship • Substance abuse • "Law" trouble • Affect • Mood • Social life • Household responsibility • Recreation • General "happiness"	Self-report 42 items	Does not include specific psychiatric symptoms
Psychological symptomatic distress identification Initial evaluation/patient progress measurement Primary Dimensional Scales: • Somatization • Depression • Anxiety • Hostility • Psychoticism • Obsessive-compulsive • Interpersonal sensitivity • Paranoid ideation • Phobic anxiety	Adult and adolescent population usage Administration time: 1 to 3 minutes Can also be used to collect outcome data	

(continued)

Product	Format	Cost	Source
Symptom Checklist-90 Revised (SCL-90-R)	Paper and pencil Computer	$2.35 each (500 minimum)	National Computer Systems, Inc. 5605 Green Circle Drive Minnetonka, MN 55343 800-627-7271
Timberlawn Child Functioning Scale (TCFS)	Paper and pencil		Dimperio, T., Blotcky, M., Gossett, J., & Doyle, A. (1985). The Timberlawn Child Functioning Scale: A preliminary report on reliability and validity. *The Psychiatric Hospital, 17*(3), 115–119.

Characteristics of Products Available for Assessment

Capabilities	Advantages	Disadvantages
90 items Multidimensional measure of psychological symptoms Level of severity measurement	Brief Self-administered Yields specific numeric scores that aid in pre- and posttesting comparisons	
Clinical assessment: • Likability • Thinking/behavior • Impulse control • Personal hygiene • Self-help skills • Adaptability • Diagnosis • Family support • Language • Attention span/activity level • Educational performance • Industry/competence • Sexuality • Acceptance of rules • Social relatedness	Appropriate for research collection data predicting long-term adjustment	

References

Agency for Health Care Policy and Research (AHCPR). (1993, April). *Depression in Primary Care: Vol. 1. Detection and Diagnosis. Clinical Practice Guideline, Number 5* (AHCPR Publication No. 93–0550). Rockville, MD: U.S. Department of Health and Human Services, Public Health Services.

Altrocchi, J., Antonuccio, D., Basta, R., & Danton, W. G. (1994). Nondrug treatment of anxiety. *American Family Physician, 10,* 161–166.

American Psychiatric Association. (1994). *Diagnostic and statistical manual of mental disorders,* (4th ed.). Washington, DC: Author.

American Psychological Association Clinical Division 12. (1993). *What is clinical psychology?* Oklahoma City, OK: Author.

American Psychological Association Practice Directorate. (1994). *APA member focus groups on the health care environment: A summary report.* Washington, DC: American Psychological Association. (800-374-2721)

Anderson, D. F., & Berlant, J. L. (1994). Managed mental health and substance abuse services. In P. R. Kongstvedt (Ed.), *The managed health care handbook* (pp. 130–140). Gathersberg, MD: Aspen.

Applebaum, P. S. (1993). Legal liability in managed care. *American Psychologist, 48*(3), 251–257.

Armstrong, S. C., & Took, K. J. (1993). Psychiatric managed care at a rural MEDDAC. *Military Medicine, 11,* 717–721.

Baldwin, J. (1995a, February). New manual to help primary care physicians diagnose mental illness. *Psychiatric Times, 11,* 29.

Baldwin, J. (1995b, February). Questionnaire helps primary care physicians detect mental disorders. *Psychiatric Times, 11,* 30.

247

Bales, J. (1987, April). A few smart habits cut malpractice risks. *APA Monitor*, 48.

Barrett, C., & Vein, C. (1995, January). Personal computing: Psychologists do and learn more—in less time. *Practitioner Focus, 3*, 10–11, 24.

Beck, A. T. (1967). *Depression: Clinical, experimental, and theoretical aspects*. New York: Hoeber.

Beck, P., Kastrup, M., & Rafaelsen, O. J. (1986). Mini-compendium of rating scales for anxiety, depression, mania, schizophrenia with corresponding *DSM-III* syndromes. *Acta Psychiatry in Scandinavia, 73*, 1–39.

Beckham, E., & Leber, W. R. (1985). *Handbook of depression: Treatment, assessment and research*. Homewood, IL: Dorsey Press.

Beetar, J. T., & Williams, J. M. (1995). Malingering response styles in the memory assessment scales and symptom validity tests. *Archives of Clinical Neuropsychology, 10*, 57–72.

Behavioral outcomes to be measured. (1994, December 2). *CCH Monitor, 2*(24), 16.

Bergeron, C. M., & Monto, G. L. (1985). Personality pattern seen in irritable bowel syndrome patients. *The American Journal of Gastroenterology, 80*, 448–451.

Bergman, R. (1994, December 20). TQM merger trailblazer? *Hospitals and Health Networks, 44*, 46.

Binder, L. M., & Pankratz, L. (1987). Neuropsychological evidence of a factitious memory complaint. *Journal of Clinical and Experimental Neuropsychology, 9*, 167–171.

Bonfils, S., & De M'Uzon, I. (1974). Irritable bowel syndrome vs. ulcerative colitis. *Journal of Psychosomatic Research, 18*, 291–296.

Borquist, L., Hansson, L., Lindelow, G., Nettlebladt, P., & Nordstrom, G. (1993). Perceived health and high consumers of care: A study of mental health problems in a Swedish health care district. *Psychological Medicine, 23*, 763–770.

Borus, J. F., & Olendzki, M. C. (1985). The offset effect of mental health treatment on ambulatory medical care utilization and charges. *Archives of General Psychiatry, 42*, 573–580.

Brody, D. S. (1980). Physician recognition of behavioral, psychological, and social aspects of medical care. *Archives of Internal Medicine, 140*, 1286–1289.

Buffone, G. W. (1989). Consultations with oral surgeons: New roles for medical psychotherapists. *Medical Psychotherapy, 2,* 33–48.

Burke, M. (1992, March 5). Clinical quality initiatives: The search for meaningful—and accurate—measures. *Hospitals,* 26–40.

Case, T. (1995, March). TQM tools strike rich vein. *Provider, 8,* 67–69.

Cattell, H. S. (1977). The role of trait assessment in clinical medicine. In S. E. Krug (Ed.), *Psychological assessment in medicine* (pp. 11–26). Champaign, IL: Institute for Personality and Ability Testing.

Claxton, J. (1995). *Response to subpoena.* Crystal Lake, IL: Claxton & Associates.

Colby, K. M., & Colby, P. M. (1992). *Overcoming depression 2.0.* Malibu, CA: Malibu Artifactual Intelligence Works.

Committee on Professional Standards & Committee on Psychological Tests and Assessment. (1986). *Guidelines for computer-based tests and interpretations.* Washington, DC: American Psychological Association.

Couch, J. B., & Warshaw, J. B. (1993). Quality management in corporate America. In J. Couch (Ed.), *Healthcare quality management for the 21st century* (pp. 391–395). Tampa, FL: American College of Physician Executives.

Coulehan, J. L., Schulberg, H. C., & Block, M. R. (1989). The efficiency of depression questionnaires for case finding in primary medical care. *Journal of General Internal Medicine, 4,* 542–547.

Crick, G. D. (1990, March). When a psychologist is investigated. *Illinois Psychologist, 21,* 4–5.

Crosby, P. (1979). *Quality free: The art of making quality certain.* Milwaukee, WI: ASQC Quality Press.

Crosby, P. (1984). *Quality without tears.* Milwaukee, WI: ASQC Quality Press.

Cummings, N. A. (1985, August). *The new mental health care delivery system and psychology's new role.* Awards Address presented at a meeting of the American Psychological Association, Los Angeles, CA.

Cummings, N. A. (1986). The dismantling of our health system. Strategies for the survival of psychological practice. *American Psychologist, 41,* 426–431.

REFERENCES

Cummings, N. A. (1990, February). *Psychologists: An essential component to cost-effective, innovative care.* Paper presented at a meeting of the American College of Healthcare Executives, Chicago, IL.

Cummings, N. A. (1992). The future of psychotherapy: Society's charge to professional psychology. *Independent Practitioner, 12*(3), 126–130.

Cummings, N. A. (1995). Behavioral health after managed care: The next opportunity for professional psychology. *Register Report, 20*(3), 1, 30–33.

Cummings, N. A., Dorken, H., Pallak, M. S., & Henke, C. J. (1990, April). *The impact of psychological intervention on healthcare utilization and costs.* San Francisco: Biodyne Institute.

Cummings, N. A., & Follette, W. T. (1968). Psychiatric services and medical utilization in a prepaid health plan setting: Part 2. *Medical Care, 6,* 31–41.

Cummings, N. A., & Sobel, S. B. (1985). Malpractice insurance: Update on sex claims. *Psychotherapy, 22*(2), 186–188.

Derogatis, L. R. (1977). *Symptoms Checklist-90-Revised (SCL-90-R) manual.* Baltimore, MD: Clinical Psychometric Research.

Dobson, K. S. (1985). An analysis of anxiety and depression scales. *Journal of Personality Assessment, 49*(5), 522–527.

Donnelly, E. R., Murphy, D. L., & Goodwin, R. K. (1976). Cross-sectional and longitudinal comparisons of bipolar and unipolar depressed groups on the MMPI. *Journal of Consultational Clinical Psychology, 44,* 233–237.

Drum, D. J. (1995). Changes in the mental health service delivery and finance systems and resulting implications for the national register. *Register Report, 20*(3), 4, 5, 8–10.

Dua, V., & Ross, C. (1993). Psychiatric health costs of multiple personality disorder. *American Journal of Psychotherapy, 47,* 103–112.

Eastman, F. (1995, January 6). Patient questionnaire to help doctors assess mental health. *CEO Forecast, 2.*

Eber, H. W. (1977). Personality factors in preventive medicine and health maintenance. In S. E. Krug (Ed.), *Psychological assessment in medicine* (pp. 171–194). Champaign, IL: Institute for Personality and Ability Testing.

Edell, W. S., Joy, S., & Yehuda, R. (1990). Discordance between self-report and observer-rated psychopathology in borderline patients. *Journal of Personality Disorders, 4*(4), 381–390.

250

References

Eimer, B. N. (1988). The chronic pain patient: Multimodal assessment and psychotherapy. *Medical Psychotherapy, 1*, 23–40.

Eisen, S., Grob, M., & Klein, A. (1986). BASIS: The development of a self-report measure for psychiatric evaluation. *Psychiatric Hospital, 6*, 165–171.

Eisenberg, L. (1992). Treating depression and anxiety in primary care. *New England Journal of Medicine, 326*, 1080–1083.

Ellwood, P. M., Huber, M. R., & Couch, J. B. (1991). The future: Clinical outcomes management. In J. Couch (Ed.), *Health care quality management for the 21st century* (p. 469). Tampa, FL: American College of Physician Executives.

Endicott, J., & Spitzer, R. L. (1978). A diagnostic interview: The Schedule for Affective Disorders and Schizophrenia. *Archives of General Psychiatry, 35*, 837–844.

Erdman, H. P., Klein, M. H., & Greist, J. H. (1985). Direct patient computer interviewing. *Journal of Counseling and Clinical Psychology, 53*(6), 760–772.

Esler, N. E., & Goulston, K. J. (1973). Levels of anxiety in colonic disorders. *New England Journal of Medicine, 1*, 16–20.

Fee, practice, and managed care survey. (1995, January). *Psychotherapy Finances, 21*(1), 1–8.

Fiedler, J. L., & Wight, J. B. (1989). *The medical offset effect and public health policy: Mental health industry in transition.* New York: Praeger.

Fifer, S. K. (1994, September). HMO primary care physicians fail to recognize and treat anxiety disorders. *Archives of General Psychiatry, 51*, 740–750.

Follette, W. T., & Cummings, N. A. (1967). Psychiatric services and medical utilization in a prepaid health plan setting. *Medical Care, 5*, 25–35.

Franklin, J., & Williams, A. F. (1993). Annual economic costs attributable to cigarette smoking in Texas. *Texas Medicine, 89*, 56–60.

Fulop, G., Strain, J. J., Hammer, J. S., & Lyons, J. S. (1989, January). Medical disorders associated with psychiatric comorbidity and prolonged hospital stay. *Hospital and Community Psychiatry, 40*(1), 80–82.

Garfield, S. L. (1974). *Clinical psychology: The study of personality and behavior.* Chicago: Aldine.

Georgia Psychological Association. (1991). *Psychologists' role in medical cost offset* [brochure]. Atlanta, GA: Author.

Gergen, D. (1991, August 19). America's legal mess. *U.S. News & World Report*, 72.

Goebel, R. A. (1983). Detection of faking on the Halstead-Reitan neuropsychological test battery. *Journal of Clinical Psychology, 39*, 731–742.

Goldenberg, H. (1973). *Contemporary clinical psychology.* Monterey, CA: Brooks/Cole.

Goodwin, F. K., & Moskowitz, J. (1993). *Healthcare reform for Americans with severe mental illness: Report of National Advisory Mental Health Council.* Washington, DC: National Advisory Mental Health Council Publications.

Gould, R. L. (1994, September). Computer-assisted therapy. *Employee Assistance*, 22–26.

Greenfield, S. (1993). The use of outcomes in medical practice application of the Medical Outcomes Study. In J. Couch (Ed.), *Health care quality management for the 21st century* (p. 432). Tampa, FL: American College of Physician Executives.

Grinfeld, M. J. (1995, January). Outcomes conference forges new alliances. *Psychiatric Times*, 54–55.

Hamilton, M. (1968). Development of a rating scale for primary depressive illness. *British Journal of Social and Clinical Psychology, 6*, 278–296.

Hankin, J. R., Kessler, L. G., Goldberg, I. D., Steinwachs, D. M., & Starfield, B. H. (1983). A longitudinal study of offset in the use of nonpsychiatric services following specialized mental health care. *Medical Care, 21*, 1099–1110.

Heaton, R. K., Smith, H. H., Lehman, R. A. W., & Vogt, A. T. (1978). Prospects for faking believable deficits on neuropsychological testing. *Journal of Consulting and Clinical Psychology, 46*, 892–900.

Hendler, N. (1984). The chronic pain patient. In F. G. Guggenheim & M. F. Weiner (Eds.), *Manual of psychiatric consultation and emergency care.* New York: Jason Aronson.

Hersch, L., & Staunton, V. (1995). Adapting to health care reform and managed care: Three strategies for survival and growth. *Professional Psychology: Research and Practice, 26*(1), 16–26.

Hinton, J. A., & Stout, C. E. (1992). Patient satisfaction. In M. B. Squire, C. E. Stout, & D. H. Ruben (Eds.), *Current advances in inpatient care.* Westport, CT: Greenwood Press.

References

Hiscock, M., & Hiscock, C. K. (1989). Refining the forced-choice method for the detection of malingering. *Journal of Clinical and Experimental Neuropsychology, 11*, 967–974.

Holder, H. D., & Blose, J. O. (1987). Changes in health care costs and utilization associated with mental health treatment. *Hospital and Community Psychiatry, 38*, 1070–1075.

Howick & Gray. (1992). *Team Member Training for Continuous Improvement manual.* Chicago: University of Chicago.

Inman, L. (1981). *The cost-effectiveness of psychotherapy.* Paper presented at a meeting of the 1981–1982 NCPA Insurance Committee.

Jacobs, D. F. (1987). Cost-effectiveness of specialized psychological programs for reducing hospital stays and outpatient visits. *Journal of Clinical Psychology, 43*, 729–735.

Jencks, S. F. (1985). Recognition of mental distress and diagnosis of mental disorders in primary care. *Journal of the American Medical Association, 253*, 1903–1907.

Joint Commission on Accreditation of Healthcare Organizations. (1991). *Transitions: From QA to CQI.* Oak Brook Terrace, IL: Author.

Jones, K. (Ed.). (1979). Report of a conference on the impact of alcohol, drug abuse, and mental health treatment on medical care utilization. *Medical Care, 17*(Suppl.), 1–82.

Jones, M. M. (1989). Multimodal treatment of irritable bowel syndrome. *Medical Psychotherapy, 2*, 12–20.

Kelleher, K. (June, 1995). Mental health in primary care: Major trends and issues. *Policy in Perspective, 1*, 3–4.

Kerlinger, F. H. (1973). *Foundations of behavioral research.* New York: Holt, Rinehart and Winston.

Kessler, L. G., Cleary, P. G., & Burke, J. D. (1985). Psychiatric disorders in primary care. *Archives of General Psychiatry, 42*, 583–587.

Kessler, L. G., Steinwachs, D. M., & Hankin, J. R. (1982). Episodes of psychiatric care and medical utilization. *Medical Care, 20*, 1209–1221.

Kiser, L. J., Wagner, B. D., & Knight, M. A. (1994, November/December). Quality indicators for partial hospitalization. *Behavioral Healthcare Tomorrow, 3*, 31–35.

Kline, D. (1995, February). Multimedia gets real. *Wired, 2*, 51–52.

Krug, S. E. (Ed.). (1977). *Psychological assessment in medicine.* Champaign, IL: Institute for Personality and Ability Testing.

Kull, R. K. (1989, February). Risk management: Avoiding the frontal malpractice assault. *Carrier Foundation Newsletter, 140,* 1–4.

Lamson, R. J. (1995, January/February). Virtual therapy: The treatment of phobias in cyberspace. *Behavioral Healthcare Tomorrow, 5,* 51–53.

Latimer, P. R. (1983). *Functional gastrointestinal disorders.* New York: Springer.

Lazarus, A. A. (1981). *The practice of multimodal therapy: Systematic, comprehensive, and effective psychotherapy.* New York: McGraw-Hill.

Lechnyr, R. (1992). Cost savings and effectiveness of mental health services. *Journal of the Oregon Psychological Association, 38,* 8–12.

Lechnyr, R. (1993). The cost savings of mental health services. *EAP Digest, 4,* 22–23.

Lumry, A. E. (1978). *Bipolar Affective Disorder: A clinical genetic study.* Unpublished doctoral dissertation, University of Minnesota, Minneapolis.

Lyons, J. S., Hammer, J. S., Strain, J. J., & Fulop, G. (1986). The timing of psychiatric consultation in general hospital and length of hospital stay. *General Hospital Psychiatry, 8,* 159–162.

Managed care: How important is outcomes research to payors? (1995, February 7). *Psychotherapy Finances, 21*(2), Issue 250, 1.

Marsella, J., Hirschfeld, R., & Katz, M. (1987). *The measurement of depression.* New York: Guilford Press.

Maruish, M. (1991). Continuous quality improvement and mental health service delivery. *Assessment Applications, 4,* 7–8.

Massad, P., West, A., & Friedman, M. (1990). Relationship between utilization of mental health and medical services in a VA hospital. *American Journal of Psychiatry, 147,* 465–469.

Matarazzo, J. D. (1992). Psychological testing and assessment in the 21st Century. *American Psychologist, 147,* 1007–1018.

McCarthy, K. (1995, February). Psychologists help quell anguish of the ill. *APA Monitor,* 10–11.

McGrady, B. S. (1986). Cost effectiveness of alcoholism treatment in partial hospital versus inpatient settings after brief inpatient treatment: 12 month outcomes. *Journal of Consulting and Clinical Psychology, 54,* 708–713.

References

Melzack, R. (1975). The McGill Pain Questionnaire: Major properties and scoring methods. *Pain, 1*, 277–299.

Meszaros, E. (1994). Looking beyond Fox v. Healthnet. *Managed Healthcare, 4*(3), 1, 12.

Montgomery, S. A., & Asberg, M. (1979). A new depression scale designed to be sensitive to change. *British Journal of Psychiatry, 134*, 382–389.

Mumford, E., Schlesinger, H. J., & Glass, G. V. (1982). The effects of psychological intervention on recovery from surgery and heart attacks: An analysis of the literature. *American Journal of Public Health, 72*, 141–151.

Mumford, E., Schlesinger, H., Glass, G., Patrick, C., & Cuerdon, T. (1984). A new look at evidence about reduced cost of medical utilization following mental health treatment. *American Journal of Psychiatry, 141*, 1145–1158.

Murphy, J. (1995, March). Grateful Med: An easy on-line tap into the National Library of Medicine. *Group Practice Managed Healthcare News, 30*, 36.

Nakamura, K., Tanaka, A., & Takano, T. (1993). The social cost of alcohol abuse in Japan. *Journal of the Studies of Alcohol, 5*, 618–625.

National Association of Psychiatric Health Systems. (1994). *Annual survey, 1993*. Washington, DC: Author.

National Cancer Center for Health Statistics. (1993). Advance report on final mortality statistics, 1991. *Monthly Vital Statistics Report, 42*(2), 5.

National Committee for Quality Assurance. (1993, October). *HEDIS 2.0: Executive summary*. Washington, DC: Author.

National Computer Systems. (1995). *Product catalog*. Minnetonka, MN: Author.

Neal, W. L. (1977). Office psychiatry for the primary care physician. In S. E. Krug (Ed.), *Psychological assessment in medicine* (pp. 27–62). Champaign, IL: Institute for Personality and Ability Testing.

Negley, E. T. (1985). Malpractice and risk management. In P. A. Kellar & L. O. Ritt (Eds.), *Innovations in clinical practice* (pp. 243–251). Sarasota, FL: PRE.

Office of the Inspector General. (1993). *Hospital incentives to physicians* (pp. 1–2). Washington, DC: U.S. Department of Health and Human Services.

REFERENCES

O'Kane, M. E. (1993). Outside accreditation of managed care plans. In P. R. Kongstvedt (Ed.), *The managed health care handbook* (pp. 231–244). Gathersberg, MD: Aspen.

Orleans, C. T., George, L. K., Houpt, J. L., & Brodie, H. (1985). How primary care physicians treat psychiatric disorders: A national survey of family practitioners. *American Journal of Psychiatry, 142,* 52–57.

Panzarino, P. J., & Kellar, J. (1994, November/December). Integrating outcomes, quality and utilization data for profiling behavioral health providers. *Behavioral Health Care Tomorrow, 4,* 27–30.

Piotrowski, C. (1984). The status of projective techniques: Or "wishing won't make it go away." *Journal of Clinical Psychology, 40,* 1495–1502.

Piotrowski, C., & Keller, J. W. (1984). Psychodiagnostic testing in APA-approved clinical psychology programs. *Professional Psychology: Research and Practice, 15,* 450–456.

Piotrowski, C., & Zalewski, C. (1993). Training in psychodiagnostic testing in APA-approved, Psy.D. and Ph.D. clinical psychology programs. *Journal of Personality Assessment, 61,* 394–405.

Pope, K., & Vasquez, M. (1991). *Ethics in psychotherapy and counseling: A practical guide for psychologists.* San Francisco: Jossey-Bass.

Popkin, M. K. (1993). "Secondary" syndromes in *DSM-IV:* A review of the literature. In A. J. Frances & T. Widiger (Eds.), *DSM-IV sourcebook.* Washington, DC: American Psychiatric Press.

Pruitt, J. A., Smith, M. C., Thelen, M. H., & Lubin, B. (1985). Attitudes of academic clinical psychologists toward projective techniques: 1968–1983. *Professional Psychology: Research and Practice, 16,* 781–788.

Price, D. P., & Cisco, A. (1985). The economic costs of alcohol and drug abuse and mental illness. *Medical Care, 23,* 109–111.

Psychotherapy Finances. (1994, April). If a suit is filed. *Psychotherapy Finances,* 7–8.

Quale, D. (1993, May 27). Clinton is right on tort problem, wrong on solution. *Wall Street Journal,* p. A24.

Regier, D. A., Narrow, W. E., & Rae, D. S. (1993). The de facto U.S. Mental and Addictive Disorders Service System: Epidemiologic catchment area perspective. *Archives of General Psychiatry, 50,* 85–94.

Rey, A. (1941). L'examen psychologique dans le cas d'encephalopathie traumatique. *Archives de Psychologie, 37,* 126–139.

Rey, A. (1964). *L'examen Clinique en Psychologie*. Paris: Presses Universitaires de France.

Richter, J. E., Obrecht, W. F., & Laurence, A. B. (1986). Psychological comparison of patients with nutcracker esophagus and irritable bowel syndrome. *Digestive Diseases and Sciences, 31*(2), 131–138.

Rosenfeld, J. P., Ellwanger, J., & Sweet, J. (in press). Detecting simulated amnesia with event-related brain potentials. *International Journal of Psychophysiology*.

Ross, R. (1995, February). Fashionable computing: PC wear in 2005. *PC World*, 54–55.

Rush, A. J., Guiles, D. E., Schledder, M. A., Fulton, C. L., Weissenberger, J., & Burns, C. (1986). The Inventory for Depressive Symptomology (IDS): Preliminary findings. *Psychiatry Research, 18*, 65–87.

Sandler, R. S., Drossman, D. A., Nathan, H. P., & McKee, D. C. (1984). Symptom complaints and health care seeking behavior in subjects with bowel dysfunction. *Gastroenterology, 87*, 314–318.

Schlesinger, H. J., Mumford, E., Glass, G., Patrick, C., & Sharfstein, S. (1983). Mental health treatment and medical care utilization in a fee-for-service system: Outpatient mental health treatment following the onset of a chronic illness. *American Journal of Public Health, 73*, 422–429.

Schmitting, G. (Ed.). (1993). *Facts about family practice*. Kansas City, MO: American Academy of Family Physicians.

Schoech, D., & Smith, K. K. (1995, January/February). Use of electronic networking for the enhancement of mental health services. *Behavioral Healthcare Tomorrow, 5*, 23–29.

Schulberg, H. C., Saul, M., McClelland, M. M., Ganguli, M., Christy, W., & Frank, R. (1985). Assessing depression in primary medical and psychiatric practices. *Archives of General Psychiatry, 42*, 1164–1170.

Selmi, P. M. (1983). *Cognitive-behavior therapy for depression 2.0*. Madison: University of Wisconsin, Department of Psychiatry.

Selmi, P. M., Klein, M. H., Griest, J. H., Sorrell, S. P., & Erdman, H. P. (1990). Computer-assisted cognitive therapy for depression. *American Journal of Psychiatry, 147*(1), 51–56.

Sharfstein, S. S., Muszynski, S., & Arnett, G. M. (1984, October). Dispelling myths about mental health benefits. *Business and Health*, 7–11.

REFERENCES

Shemo, J. (1985–1986). Cost effectiveness of providing mental health services: The offset effect. *International Journal of Psychiatry in Medicine, 15*, 19–30.

Shewhart, W. A. (1939). *Statistical methods from the viewpoint of quality control* (p. 7). Washington, DC: U.S. Department of Agriculture Graduate School.

Shipley, R. H., Orleans, C. T., Wilbur, C. S., Piserchia, P., & McFadden, D. (1988). Effect of Johnson & Johnson Live for Life Program on employee smoking. *Preventive Medicine, 17*, 25–34.

Shumaker, R. G. (1990). Orienting the physician-referred patient to psychological intervention. *Medical Psychotherapy, 3*, 141–146.

Silver, R. J., Isaacs, K., & Mansky, P. (1981). MMPI correlates of affective disorders. *Journal of Clinical Psychology, 31*, 836–839.

Slack, W. V., & Slack, C. W. (1977). Talking to a computer about emotional problems: A comparative study. *Psychotherapy: Theory, Research, and Practice, 14*(2), 156–163.

Soisson, E. L., VandeCreek, L., & Knapp, S. (1987). Thorough record keeping. *Professional Psychology, 18*(5), 498–502.

Spitzer, R. L., Williams, J. B. W., Kroenke, K., Linzer, M., Verloin deGruy, F., Hahn, S. R., & Brody, D. (1994a). Primary Care Evaluation of Mental Disorders (PRIME●MD) manual. New York: Biometrics Research.

Spitzer, R. L., Williams, J. B. W., Kroenke, K., Linzer, M., Verloin deGruy, F., Hahn, S. R., & Brody, D. (1994b, December 14). Utility of a new procedure for diagnosing mental disorders in primary care: The PRIME●MD study. *Journal of the American Medical Association, 272*(22), 1749–1756.

Stair, T. (1995, January). Preventive health & wellness programs to increase. *Open Minds, 6*, 12.

Stout, C. E. (1988). A clinician's guide to differential diagnosis between physical and psychiatric disorders. *Medical Psychotherapy, 1*, 65–72.

Stout, C. E. (1989). A methodological approach to differential diagnostics. In K. Anchor (Ed.), *The handbook of medical psychotherapy: Cost-effective strategies in mental health* (pp. 139–150). Lewiston, NY: Hogrefe & Huber.

Stout, C. E. (1990). Software development for the non-programmer: An instructional clinical example. *Behavioral Research Methods, Instruments, and Computers, 22*(2), 200–201.

Stout, C. E. (1994). The differential diagnosis of psychological symptoms. In L. F. Koziol & C. E. Stout (Eds.), *The neuropsychology of mental disorders* (pp. 32–38). Springfield, IL: Charles C. Thomas.

Stout, C. E. (in press). Automated methods of clinical quality management. In M. Miller, M. Hile, & K. Hammond (Eds.), *Mental health computing*. New York: Springer-Verlag.

Stout, C. E., Thies, G., & Oher, J. (Eds.). (1996). *The complete guide to managed behavioral care*. New York: Wiley.

Stromberg, C., & Dellinger, A. (1993, December). Malpractice and other professional liability. *The Psychologist's Legal Update* [newsletter].

Strumwasser, I., Paranjpe, N. V., Udow, M., Share, D., Wisgerhof, M., Ronis, D. L., Bartzack, C., & Saad, A. N. (1991, August). Appropriateness of psychiatric and substance abuse hospitalization: Implications for payment and utilization management. *Medical Care, 29*(Suppl.), AS77–AS90.

Sundberg, N. D. (1961). The practice of psychological testing in clinical services in the United States. *American Psychologist, 16,* 79–83.

Tearnan, B. H., & Lewandowski, M. J. (1992). Behavioral assessment of pain. *American Journal of Pain Management, 20*(4), 181–191.

Theis, G., Geraty, R., Panzarino, P., & Bartlett, J. (1995, March). Toward the behavioral health report card. *Medical Interface, 20,* 2–5.

Thelen, M. H., Varble, D. L., & Johnson, J. (1968). Attitudes of academic clinical psychologists toward projective techniques. *American Psychologist, 23,* 517–521.

Turk, D. C., Meichenbaum, D., & Genest, M. (1983). *Pain and behavioral medicine: A cognitive-behavioral perspective*. New York: Guilford Press.

Turner, J. A., & Romano, J. M. (1984). Self-report screening measures for depression in chronic pain patients. *Journal of Clinical Psychology, 40*(4), 909–913.

VandeCreek, L., & Stout, C. E. (1993). Risk management in inpatient psychiatric care. In M. B. Squire, C. E. Stout, & D. H. Ruben (Eds.), *Current advances in inpatient psychiatric care* (pp. 53–67). Westport, CT: Greenwood Press.

VandenBos, G. R., & DeLeon, P. H. (1988). The use of psychotherapy to improve physical health. *Psychotherapy, 25,* 335–343.

Walen, J. (1985). *Use of short-term general hospitals by patients with psychiatric diagnoses* (DHHS Publication No. PHS-86-3395). Washington, DC: U.S. Government Printing Office.

Ware, J. E., Manning, W. G., Duan, N., Wells, K., & Newhouse, J. (1984). Health status and the use of outpatient mental health services. *American Psychologist, 39*, 1090–1100.

Watkins, C. E., Jr., Campbell, V. L., Nieberding, R., & Hallmark, R. (1995). Contemporary practice of psychological assessment by clinical psychologists. *Professional Psychology: Research and Practice, 26*(1), 54–60.

Watson, R. I. (1953). A brief history of clinical psychology. *Psychological Bulletin, 50*, 321–346.

Weizenbaum, J. (1966). ELIZA—A computer program for the study of natural language communication between man and machine. *Communications of the Association for Computer Machinery, 9*, 36–45.

Wells, K. B., Stewart, A., Hays, R. D., Burham, M. A., Rogers, W., Daniels, M., Berry, S., Greenfield, S., & Ware, J. (1989). Detection of depressive disorder for patients receiving prepaid or fee-for-service care. *Journal of the American Medical Association, 262*, 3298–3302.

Werkman, S. L., Mallory, J., & Harris, J. (1976). The common psychiatric problems in family practice. *Psychosomatics, 17*(3), 119–122.

Whitted, B. (1990). Vicarious liability: Psychologist acting as supervisor. *Illinois Psychologist, 21*, 2–4.

Wiggins, J. G., Jr. (1994). Would you want your child to be a psychologist? *American Psychologist, 49*(6), 485–492.

Williams, J. M. (1991). *Memory assessment scales.* Odessa, FL: Psychological Assessment Resources.

Wing, J., Birley, J., Cooper, J., Graham, P., & Isaacs, A. (1967). Reliability of a procedure for measuring and classifying "Present Psychiatric State." *British Journal of Psychiatry, 113*, 499–515.

Yates, B. T. (1984). How psychology can improve effectiveness an reduce costs of health services. *Psychotherapy, 21*, 439–451.

Zappia, P., & Watrons, J. (1995, January/February). Designing and integrated, initial patient assessment. *Joint Commission Perspectives,* 13–15.

Author Index

261

Author Index

Subject Index